INEQUALITIES IN UNDERSERVED COMMUNITIES- A PUBLIC HEALTH PERSPECTIVE AND IN COVID19

Inequalities In Underserved Communities- A Public Health Perspective and in COVID19

Impact of Bad Public Policy
on Certain Population

Chuks A. Iregbu

To order additional copies of this book, contact:
Xlibris
844-714-8691
www.Xlibris.com
Orders@Xlibris.com
828205

Contents

PREFACE

How can a public health professional explain what the term public health mean in a lay person's language? It may not seem that simple. However, all efforts must show how every day human activities and interactions among people in different communities are affected by public policy. More importantly, it must express how public health means the holistic wellbeing of everyone in the society. This book came to be as a matter of concern on how some people go through various difficult times created by others in other to exist. Indeed, some individuals in a society consistently make live more uncomfortable for others either by their direct or indirect actions. Inequalities in life among human society is seen by some people as a norm while others grumble about it. In a democratic society, citizens assume freedom with the expectations that having representatives they elected by a majority vote will protect their interests. All things being equal, such expectation is supposed to hold. The irony is that some elected officials representing and expected to protect and fight for the interest of those who voted them into office turn their back to pursue a different and personal interest.

The scope of this book will avoid inclusion of elaborate technical data but will provide and expand on facts and points relevant to the purpose of writing the book. That is, how and why the common person and those on the economic bottom continue to struggle to survive in the society. The book also looked into how epidemiology is viewed by scholars and the role it plays in public health. It further integrated epidemiology with evidence-based studies that shape public health policies. It also addressed the importance of epidemiology relative to morbidity and mortality among different population. Other highlights include education of the general public on how a disease outbreak can be controlled providing information for decision making to protect human population. Nonetheless, such information does not automatically imply a provision for safety on diseases or risk factors rather it must be reviewed, analysed and weighed against economic, social and environmental health determinants for policy formation.

In addition, the book pointed out that new disease outbreak symptoms, diagnosis and treatment can be different and may require non-existing drug(s) for effective treatment. Such scenario invokes vaccine research with acceptable efficacy and limited adverse effect. This requires rigorous efforts including funding, time and volunteers for clinical trials. These variables must be at optimum values as to minimize public bias. Finally it showed how COVID19 mortality rate held same pattern of impact as other diseases and natural disasters on the less affluent population.

Acknowledgment

The author would like to thank his wife and children for their encouragement, moral and other supports, and accommodating his absence of attention during the process of writing and publishing this book. The author further expressed his appreciation to Dr. Henry Kerich a fellow professor at Strayer University for his profound professional and inspirational gesturers in choosing the ultimate publisher.

DEDICATION

The author dedicate this book to his late older brother Robinson A. Iregbu-Nwogu, popularly known as Chief Eze Omenma. He regrets that Chief Eze Omenma Robinson Nwogu who played the role of best friend, brother and father to him did not live long enough to read the book.

CHAPTER 1

Why You May Not Be Protected In the Public Health Arena

Hidden Agenda in Public Policy

Every prospective political candidate aspiring for an elective political position at a local, state or national level will play a frank intension to serve his or her political constituent to the best of their benefit. While some voters remain in a contemplation stage on who to vote in as the campaign communication intensify, others have their mind fixed on who should represent them. The fact is that the majority of the voters fall into the psychological permutation for choice of the right candidate. Nonetheless, the desire is the need to have a representative that will stand firm to protect the population that voted him or her in. We have often heard that politicians are not honest, putting it in the mildest form. This may be an assumption without valid research to back it up. On the other hand, the action of some elected officials at the long run tend to support this notion well. One thing that is becoming obvious is that we are all politicians at our own levels at different times. Most people tend to promise to impress others without solid resources backing to fulfil what they promised. As the dynamics of events follow, those promises begin to evaporate.

At political arena and constituencies the inability to deliver turns to become defensive challenges. Some supporters tend to grant mercy but others see it as abandonment especially the less privileged. Political insiders know why some of the promises fell short or get put in back burner. Affluent interest groups invest excess efforts in dissuading elected officials to vote against legislation that protect and benefit the common people. This is a huge factor that many voters and or supporters across the country do not comprehend. It has become obvious that most of the officials we vote into the house of representative and senate alike in all forms of government level; local, state and federal succumb to the social behavioral theory of expectancy-value (EV) theory. This is a behavior theory that implicates the tendency of human attraction to rewarding temptations contrary to more appropriate moral and ethical considerations. This means people tend to behave and act upon conditions under which they can most likely predict the likelihood of an attractive future outcome (Wigfield, & Eccles, 2000). In this concept they have already made up their mind on how to vote on a public policy that may affect the public health (Sutton, McVey & Glanz, 1999).

One disturbing fact is that in applying expectancy theory based on various research findings, those acting under such influence fail to consider the consequences of their specific actions and decisions. Rather what they relate to is only the expected value outcome to their own gratuity (Frankish, Lovato, & Shannon, 1999). While some people tend to uphold their innermost honesty, the weakness of the mind falls a prey to comparative peer pressure from their colleagues who has preconceived a reward of value in tangible or intangible form. Knowing that value(s) is a conceptual relationship between anticipated rewards that gratifies one as a suitable substitute for something else. Feather (1992) analyzed values and motives with the assumption that value acts as a function of motives in that the value people attribute to an action influences their drive to pursue goal-directed activities. Nonetheless, the level of activities depends on certain factors that include effort invested in the activities, duration of activities, and persistence of the activities (Feather, 1992).

Expectancy value theory is more suitable for this chapter and section of this book because other behavioral theories and constructs, such as diffusion of innovation, involves the use of role model, learning ability, cognitive ability, developmental stages, and self-efficacy. The theory of reasoned action (TRA) embraces behavior, consequences, and values, but it is not suitable for the purpose of this public health focused piece because the construct is built around social norms. According to Frankish, Lovato, and Shannon (1999), TRA is specific to cognitive and attitude-based behavior subjected to social norms among the desires of related groups. In a study to determine how TRA played a role in affirmative action programs, Bell, Harrison, and McLaughlin (2000) concluded that attitude and subjective norms determined actions. Here, the subjective norm of intentions is predictive of reasoned action and behavior (Sutton, McVey, & Glanz, 1999). Therefore, the subject norm of intentions may not be applicable in the public policy attitudes that drive elected officials to differ from expectations, motives, and trade-off basis for the value of expectancy, internal desire and fulfilment of self-interests.

Personal versus Public Interest

As this chapter continue to drill for answer and solution into why some public policies are skewed abandoning the good intensions of democratic principles, it is reasonable to explore all the rationales positive or negative that warrants deviation from protecting the population a policy is presumed to protect. Expectancy value as an important theoretical framework for reference and construct. Moreover, it implicates some reasons why people deviate from positive norms whether in political, public policy and public health arenas. Such reasons include that:

1. Values drive people to react differently when important values are challenged.
2. People usually dislike being confronted with difficult moral choices, especially if such choices are associated with inter-group conflict for satisfying and fulfilling their values (Feather, 1992).
3. Individuals tend to accept and get involved in activities that have the potential to protect them against a strong threat (Jonas, 1993).
4. People tend to accept trade-offs between different dimensions for a high comfort level (Jonas, 1993).
5. Individuals and interest groups are more receptive to changes in programs that reflect their values and attitudes despite popular public opinions (Perlstadt, & Holmes, 1987), (Gallup, March 1-15, 2021) as seen and in attribute among members of 116th congress. This was determined in the expectancy-value model of receptivity (Wilmoth, Silver & Severy, 1987).

Not only does pre-contemplation to making decision and accepting the action dominate the individual's mind in making the choice for self-satisfaction, there is also an after effect of guilt and defensive stand to justify the wrong path followed. Feather (1992) said that motives of involvement in activities are driving forces to manipulate situations and feelings in a bidirectional mode of either successful or unsuccessful outcomes based on preset standards. Feather (1992) also articulated that values are embraced and integrated at various social institutions in such a way that different values fall under different categories based on the importance or value of the system. For example, circumstances for promulgating the residential lead-based paint disclosure policy have some value attributes. This example means that values play a role in peoples' actions even at the institutional level and in policy discourse. Knestrick & Milstead (1998) implicated the issue of values and valences in their analysis of Title X: The Residential Lead-Based Paint Hazard Reduction Act of 1992. Another example could be drawn from how the 115th and 116th congress voted for approval of the different segments of the Covid-19 pandemic relief budget package. Many elected members of the congress voted to deny or reduce the money meant to benefit and alleviate the hardship for the poor low income people. Rather, such lawmakers nodded for the package going to the rich and wealthy through tactical legislative arguments and loopholes making. Such maneuvers and presumptive interests mounted high tension for tight vote (Marcos, 2021).

It has become intricate for elected officials in many society to delineate themselves socially from this behavioral theory of expectancy-value. People tend to behave and act upon conditions under which they can most likely predict the likelihood of an attractive future outcome (Wigfield & Eccles, 2000). In applying EV theory to this piece of observation it is obvious that consequences of specific actions and decisions that our leaders make most of the time are common and related to expected value outcome that will benefit them (Frankish, Lovato & Shannon, 1999). In EV-related studies, investigators define the word "values" based on the conceptual relationship between the research problem and anticipated values. This book and chapter define *value* as a tangible or intangible subject or reward that gratifies one as a suitable substitute for something else. Feather (1992) analyzed values and motives with the assumption that value acts as a function of motives in that the value people attribute to an action influences their drive to pursue goal-directed activities. Nonetheless, the level of activities depends on certain factors that include effort invested in the activities, duration of activities, and persistence of the activities (Feather, 1992). This is indicative to why many elected officials will not like to resign from a position and will fight as hard as they must as to retain their elected offices.

Chapter One References

1. Bell, M. P., Harrison, D. A., & McLaughlin, M. E. (2000). Forming, changing, and acting on attitude toward affirmative action programs in employment: A theory-driven approach. *Journal of Applied Psychology, 85* (5), 784-798.
2. Feather, N.T. (1992). Values, Valences, Expectations, and Actions. Journal of Social Issues Volume 48, Issue 2 p. 109-124.
3. Frankish, C. J., Lovato, C.Y., & Shannon, W. J. (1999). Models, theories, and principles of health promotion with multicultural population. In Huff, R. M., & Kline, M. V. (Eds.) *Promoting health in multicultural populations: A handbook for practitioners.* Thousand Oaks, CA: Sage Publications, Inc.
4. Gallup, (2021). Congress and the Public: Congressional Job Approval, March 1-15, 2021.
5. Jonas, K. (1993). Expectancy value models of health behavior: An analysis conjoint measurement. *European Journal of Social Psychology, 23* (2), 167-183.
6. Knestrick, J., & Milstead, J. A. 1998). Public policy and child lead poisoning: Implementation of Title X. *Pediatric Nursing, 24* (1), 37-48.
7. Marcos, C. (2021). House set for tight vote on COVID-19 relief package. The Hill: 02/26/21 07:42 PM EST. Retrieved from https://thehill.com/homenews/house/540773-house-set-to-vote-on-covid-19-relief.
8. Perlstadt, H & Holmes, R. E. (1987). The role of public opinion polling in health legislation. American Journal of Public Health, 77(5), 612-614.
9. Sutton, S., McVey, D., & Glanz, A. (1999). Comparative test of the theory of reasoned action and the theory of planned behavior in the prediction of condom use intentions in a national sample of English young people. *Health Psychology, 18* (1), 72-81.

10. Wigfield, A., & Eccles, J. S. (2000). Expectancy-value theory of achievement motivation. *Contemporary Educational Psychology, 25* (9), 68-81.

11. Wilmoth, G. H., Silver, S., & Severy, L. J. (1987). Receptivity and planned change: Community attitudes and deinstitutionalization. *Journal of Applied Psychology, 72* (1), 138-145.

CHAPTER 2

What Is Bad Public Health Policy

The Lead-based Paint Policy

In a democratic government where there are checks and balances, one would expect policies that relate to the health of the citizens will have true human sensitivity. To the contrary, many times party politics comes into play to make some spoils. When the federal government stepped up its efforts to eliminate the risk of childhood lead poisoning through grants for lead paint abatement, blood screening (Kaufmann, Clouse, Olsen & Matte, 2000) and other preventive programs, opponents of the policy argued that screening fewer children would reduce the number of identified lead risk areas and thereby save the government money (Knestrick & Milstead, 1998). Similarly, during peak incidences of COVID-19 pandemic some politicians called to limit COVID-19 testing. They reasoned that limiting testing was needed as to lower case rate. The irony is that such ideology is contrary to epidemiological principles. Referencing back to the disclosure policy as an offspring of Title X seemed to satisfy the interests of the opposing group. It is obvious that if evidence based study determines that there is a correlation between decrease in the number of abatements performed and the disclosure rule, then the proponents of the policy should look into the policy again because such interest undermines the common good (Iregbu, 2011).

Trade-offs and receptivity models in expectancy-value theory have been tested in some studies, but are beyond the scope of this book. Trade-offs and receptivity models motivates and invokes interest in expectancy-value. This becomes applicable to property owners. The disclosure policy served their interests. It provided an option not to abate or pay for lead abatement and other lead-based paint risk-reductions on housing units before leasing or selling a property. A property owner may only give the potential renter or buyer a copy of the disclosure policy (the right-to-know booklet) on residential lead paint.

With this the property owner is without any binding obligation at that point before the contract is signed. Property owners seem satisfied with the rule especially those who own properties in communities where property values depreciate. This comfort of non-liability is with total disregard to lead-contaiminated house dust and effect such has on the health of children in families that will occupy the property (Lanphear, et al, 1998). Properties in low-income communities do not attract maintenance. As such, choosing not to perform lead abatements in low-income urban communities served as a trade-off that many property owners expected and valued. The conceptual framework of the expectancy-value theory was applicable in a study involving mothers in a biweekly lead-dust cleaning environment aimed at preventing lead exposure in inner-city children (Rhoads, 1998), (Charney, Kessler, Farfel & Jackson, 1983). Parents who participated in the study were motivated because of an expectancy reward of lower lead dust load in their homes and a drop in blood lead in their children.

Many times, I practically drew this issue before different cohorts of students in my healthcare administration, public health or environment science class. Topics such as health disparity and environmental health injustice in urban dwelling invoke these issues.

On explaining the expectancy-value theory to the class relative to some public health policies, I could observe discomforts in many students' faces. These could have been those who either have experienced same situation or knew someone who had no choice than to move in a non-lead abated houses just as to have a shelter. This was in no doubt a bad public policy that up till today has a negative impact on the citizens especially children of economically disadvantaged families.

Norplant Issue

One other example of bad public health policy application was when a new contraceptive that hit the market in 1991 was embraced as a new innovation to slow down teenage pregnancy in the United States. The new product was known as Norplant System (levonorgestrel) Implants. The contraceptive was manufactured and distributed by the American Home Products Corporation Maker (NYTNS, 1999). What could have been the challenges of this new product was not deeply studied. Rather, it became a measure to control fertility particularly for the underserved population (Lynn & Holdcroft, 1992). Some specific circumstances include cases where young mothers receiving government assistance were persuaded to submit to have the implant in order to continue receiving their social benefits or lose it. Others were compelled by judges to receive the implant as a check of their ability to raising children properly as an option for probation (Burrell, 1995). Here the protection of public health was not considered (Annas, 1999). One would ask whether this option would apply if the young mothers were economically independent without government financial assistance (Breiner, Ford & Gadsden, 2016).

Norplant is no longer marketed or available in the United States. Nonetheless, the sad part and irony of the issue was that many young women who were directly or indirectly compelled and received the implant experienced some unnecessary side effects (Dugoff et al., 1995). Some documented side effects include breast discharge, abdominal discomfort, cervicitis, leucorrhea, musculoskeletal pain and vaginitis among 5% or greater of the subjects during the clinical trials and first year of treatment (Cunha, n.d.). Despite these noted side effects, the product was still marketed. More so, in post marketing of the product those who used the contraceptive reported many adverse reactions or side effects (see table 2.1)

Table 2.1: Reported Adverse Reactions Post-marketing

Percentage of Victims (1%)	Adverse Reactions
	a. Arm pain. b. Gallbladder disease. c. Hypertension. d. Idiopathic intracranial hypertension (IIH) (pseudotumor cerebri, benign intracranial hypertension). e. Insertion/removal site reactions including abscess, cellulitis; blistering; bruising; edema; excessive scarring; hyperpigmentation; induration; nerve injury; numbness; sloughing; tingling. f. Ulcerations. g. Migraine headaches. h. Ovarian cysts. i. Phlebitis.

Source: American College of Osteopathic
Emergency Physicians (ACOEP).

Other side effect as documented by some studies are shown in the (table 2.2). These uncomfortable side effects drove most of the subjects to demand removal of the implant (Opara et al., 1997).

Issue	Percentage of Victims
Many bleeding days or prolonged bleeding	27.6
Spotting	17.1
Amenorrhea (*missed at least three menstrual periods*)	9.4
Irregular (onsets of) bleeding	7.6
Frequent bleeding onsets	7.0
Scanty bleeding	5.2
Pain or itching near implant site (usually transient)	3.7
Infection at implant site	0.7

Table 2.2: Some Side Effects of Norplant (levonorgestrel)
Sources: American College of Osteopathic
Emergency Physicians (ACOEP).

Although this chapter and book is not directed to elaborate on the pharmaceutical or regulatory aspect of Norplant® and Jadelle® (levonorgestrel) implants rather it is directing attention on how bad public health policy and judgments play negative roles towards the good health of others (Stein, 1999). Most unfortunately, how people at higher authorities with power of making decision that affect others proceed without consideration of the vulnerable citizens that will bear the impact of the negative health effect.

It is obvious that the judge in question (Burrell, 1995) did not consider the side effect of the product. To implement the procedure medically a trained health-care professional must be familiar with the technique on how to insert the implants. It must contain a set of two flexible cylindrical implants, each containing 75 mg of the progestin levonorgestrel. The total administered (implanted) dose is 150 mg and the two pieces must be inserted or administered during the first 7 days following the start of the recipient menses. Not only that receiving the implant by the targeted population was persuasive, they were left without any other choice if they wanted to continue receiving government assistance. Despite such pressure to submit to this birth control device, this implant subjects mostly teenage girls (Mashburn, 1994) were considered to have directly or indirectly consented to the treatment. The insertion must be subdermal (under the skin) in the midportion of the inner surface of the upper arm (Townsend, 1990). It must be positioned carefully about 8 to 10 cm above the long bone in the upper arm (medial epicondyle).

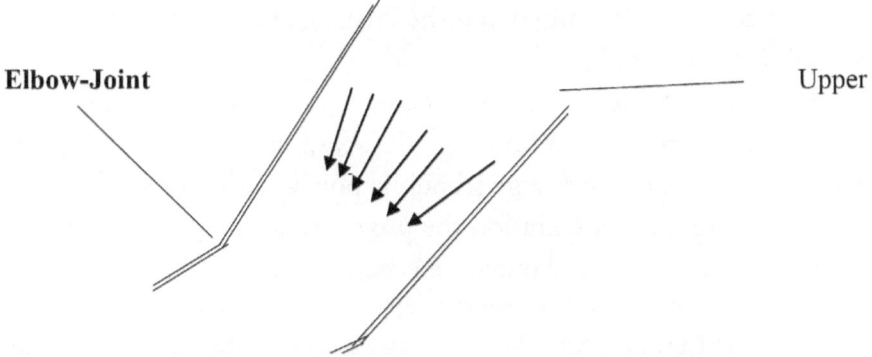

Elbow-Joint   Upper

Figure 2.1: Typical Norplant contraceptive implant inserts.

Section-8 Housing Policy.

Another area of bad public policy that impacted public health is in policy of the Federal Department of Housing and Urban Development (HUD). Public health involves the concern of protecting and improving the health of every citizen at all levels. This includes families, communities and regions of low-income or economic ladder. This can be done through promoting healthy lifestyles, advocating for various disease prevention and encouraging clean environment.

Clean environment does not exclude residential homes where families can have a sense of well-being and be safe from crimes or dangerous activities.

The core function of HUD is to facilitate affordable housing ownership for low-income citizens. This function was attached with a vision to desegregate city and urban communities. The principle aim is to enable many low-income families brake away from their long and limiting inner-city public high-rise buildings. Some of such residential complexes are commonly known as *housing projects* and they are notorious with drugs and crime activities. The opportunity for some of these families to move out and find affordable single families homes or townhouses in more affluent communities encourages desegregation. It was also designed to reduce disparities in access to health care, education and other social amenities but these outcomes were limited and the crisis of affordable housing still prevail (Crowley, 2003).

The United States Congress created a tool in 1974 to implement the plan through *Section 8* housing bill (www.baltimoresun.com). Again, one would think this was a good public policy with good intensions. However, after implementation the program need to be evaluated to determine if the intended outcome is being achieved. As both impact and outcome evaluations are necessary in any social and public health program, one would ask if any have been done on *Section 8* housing program. Evaluation is necessary especially where it is obvious that the *Section 8* program ended up limiting those who eventually qualify for communities worse than them or less much better (Samuels, 2015). The reason behind this non-progressive outcome becomes a matter of interpretation. One may ask whether the outcome is the birth of hidden agenda or it is a matter of unintended consequences (Jones & Serpas, 2016).

Chapter Two Reference

1. Annas, G.J. (1999). Burden of proof: Judging science and protecting public health in (and out of) the courtroom. American Journal of Public Health, April 1999, 89, 4, p488-486.

2. Breiner H., Ford M. & Gadsden, V.L (2016) editors. Parenting Matters: Supporting Parents of Children Ages 0-8. National Academies of Sciences, Engineering, and Medicine; Division of Behavioral and Social Sciences and Education; Board on Children, Youth, and Families; Committee on Supporting the Parents of Young Children; Washington (DC): National Academies Press (US); 2016 Nov 21.

3. Burrell, D.E., (1995). The Norplant Solution: Norplant and the Control of African-American Motherhood. UCLA Women's Law Journal 5(2). Retrieved on January 15, 2021 from https://escholarship.org/uc/item/9861n279 Journal UCLA Women's Law Journal, 5(2).

4. Charney E, Kessler B, Farfel M, Jackson D. (1983). Childhood lead poisoning. A controlled trial of the effect of dust-control measures on blood lead levels. Med. 1983;309(18):1089–93.

5. Cunha, J. P. (n.d.). Norplant Side Effects Center. American College of Osteopathic Emergency Physicians (ACOEP) Article RxList April 6, 2018.

6. Crowley, S. (2003). The affordable housing crisis: Residential mobility of poor families and school mobility of poor children. *Journal of Negro Education, 72* (1), 22-38.

7. Dugoff, L. 1; Jones, O. W. 3rd; Allen-Davis, J; Hurst, B. S. and Schlaff, W.D. (1995). Assessing the Acceptability of Norplant Contraceptive in Four Patient Populations, 1995 Jul; 52(1):45-9. doi: 10.1016/0010-7824(95)00123-r. PMID: 8521714 DOI: 10.1016/0010-7824(95)00123-r

8. Iregbu, C. A., (2008). Lead Paint Disclosure Policy: Implications for Eliminating Childhood Lead Exposure in

Baltimore City, 2008, University of Michigan Publishers. Also: Barnes and Noble Published online July 2011.

9. Jones, C. & Serpas, S. (2016). The Unintended Consequences of Housing Finance. Regional Plan Association, January 2016.

10. Kaufmann, R. B., Clouse, T. L., Olsen, D. R., & Matte, T. D. (2000). Elevated blood lead levels and blood screening among U.S. children aged one to five years: 1988-1994. *Pediatrics, 106* (6), 1472-1481.

11. Knestrick, J., & Milstead, J. A. 1998). Public policy and child lead poisoning: Implementation of Title X. *Pediatric Nursing, 24* (1), 37-48.

12. Lanphear B.P., Matte, T.D, Rogers J, et al. (1998). The contribution of lead-contaminated house dust and residential soil to children's blood lead levels. A pooled analysis of 12 epidemiologic studies. Environ Res. 1998;79(1):51–68.

13. Lynn, M.M. and Holdcroft, C.(1992). New concepts in contraception: Norplant subdermal implant. Nurse Pract. 1992 Mar;17(3):85-9. doi: 10.1097/00006205-199203000-00016. PMID: 1565306.

14. Mashburn, M. (1994). Levonorgestrel Implant Use Among Adolescents. J Pediatr Health Care, Nov-Dec 1994;8(6):255-60. doi: 10.1016/0891-5245(94)90007-8. PMID: 7799199 DOI: 10.1016/0891-5245(94)90007-8.

15. NYTNE, (1999). Norplant maker agrees to settle; 36,000 would get $1,500 each to end birth control lawsuits; A 'business decision.' NEW YORK TIMES NEWS SERVICE (NYTNS), THE BALTIMORE SUN August 27, 1999.

16. Opara, J.U.; Ernst, F.A.; Gaskin, h.; Smith, L; and Nevels, H. V. (1997). Factors Associated With Elective Norplant Removal in Black and White Women. Journal of National Medical Association. PMID: 9145628 PMCID: PMC2608206

17. Rhoads, G. G. (1998). Preventing lead exposure in inner-city children. University of Medicine and Dentistry of New

Jersey – Robert Wood Johnson Medical School, Piscataway, N.J. Retrieved from http://www.rwjf.org.

18. Samuels, A. (2015). How Housing Policy Is Failing America's Poor. The Atlantic Business News, June 24, 2015. Retrieved from: https://www.theatlantic.com /business.

19. Solaner, et al., (2014). Pinching the Poor? Medicaid Cost Sharing Under the ACA. OBSTETRICS: Ethics, Medical Issues, and Public Policy. Obstetrical & Gynecological Survey: July 2014 - Volume 69 - Issue 7 - p 384-386 doi: 10.1097/01.ogx.0000452699.74427.fc (

20. Stein, Z. A. (1999). Silicone Breast Implants: Epidemiological evidence of sequelae. American Journal of Public Health, April 1999, 89, 4, p488-486.

21. Townsend, S. (1990). Norplant Insertion and Removal. Netw Res Triangle Park N.C,1990 Dec;11(4):13-4. PMID: 12283716.

22. The U.S. House of Representatives (2010). Compilation of Patient Protection and Affordable Care Act. 111TH Congress 2d Session Office of the Legislative Counsel, May 2010.

23. Webb, B.C. (2017). Breaking Down Trump's Health Care Executive Order and the End of CSR Payments. Viewpoints – UVA Public Health Science, Monday, Oct. 9th – Friday, Oct. 13th 2017.

CHAPTER 3

Good Public Health Policy

When Interest of the People Matters

It is clear and understood that public health policies are legislated to become law or rule that must be implemented in order to benefit or affect respective groups of a population. In some instances a Presidential Executive Order (PEO) is declared by the president in terms of a national issue. At a state level, a governor can invoke a Gubernatorial Executive Order (GEO). Depending on the issue at stake either of the EOs may have impact on a specific public health policy. In contrast to the Norplant issues discussed in chapter two, one can draw an example of good public health policy to Medicaid expansion to cover children of low-income families who otherwise would have been uninsured. This was typically found in 1997 in the state of Maryland during the administration of Governor Paris N. Glendening. The then governor of the State of Maryland found an interest in a federal program that provided opportunity for a state matching fund. With that move Maryland's health coverage for uninsured children flourished (Dresser, 1997). Elsewhere and in New Jersey a good public health policy took another means to save lives. In 2005 Richard Codey as an acting Governor of the State of New Jersey utilized GEO to put regulation and monitoring for abuse of anabolic steroids among interscholastic athletes. The action was invoked from evidenced-based data of risks *of cancer, cardiovascular disease, mental health and compromise of immune, hormonal, and metabolic systems* (Gakh, et al., 2013).

Not to overstretch the issue, as Barack H. Obama, the America's 44th president and a democrat got into office, he worked hard with his democratic house and senate members to fulfil one of his core campaign promises. The promise that all Americans should have access to health care service irrespective of their economic class. The signature law of the president known as the Patient Protection Affordable Care Act (ACA) was commonly referred to as the *Obama Care*. The policy was signed into law with popular public support. One of the main clauses that attracted public support is that no American should be denied health insurance coverage based on a pre-existing condition of ill-health. This clause became effective after January 1, 2014 (Health and Human Services (HHS.gov, n.d.).

The opposite was the case prior to signing the ACA into a federal law. Then, people with pre-existing medical problems were denied a health insurance coverage or had to pay higher premiums and deductibles. For many people the financial burden becomes unbearable especially for older Americans without some kind of economic and financial security. Report and analysis by the Department of HHS indicate that approximately 19 to 50 percent of non-elderly Americans have some type of pre-existing health condition. In other words in every five non-elderly Americans one person is with a pre-existing condition and this can count for up to 25 million people (CMS.gov, n.d.). Those with financial hardship were limited from purchasing basic or extra health insurance coverage. While pre-existing medical problems' denials and discriminations prevailed, it became clear that more than 20 million Americans had no access to healthcare services. One of the consequences of such limitations was high rate of hospital emergency visits. Such emergency visits are attributed to the fact that the victims shy away in early symptoms of illness due to lack of personal physician for primary prevention and or routine check-ups.

A good public policy resonates happiness and sense of care and protection among the citizens. Hearing and seeing people protesting and asking their republican representatives "what will you replace the *Obamacare* with if you repeal it" sends a message that more people now understand the *Affordable Care Act* than ever before (Cohn, 2020). In the insurance business, some schools of thought and experts see health insurance purchase as a poll of investment by diverse population to protect individuals in case of illness. Particularly, it also serve for preventive medical check-ups. While some people may not utilize the benefit of the coverage often especially those in good health some others use the benefit frequently. It is this group of people that will be affected if the core principles of the *Affordable Care Act* are taken away. The COVID19 pandemic has thought many politicians and legislatures who seem to be pragmatics a big lessons on the need for better public health policy. This is especially seen in the states that sued the federal government seeking to invalidate the ACA (NCSL, 2017).

Citizens Well Being and Power Politics

In 2017 the 45th Presidential invoked an Executive Order to halt the Cost Sharing Reduction (CSR) for insurance premium and deductibles through federal government subsidies (Webb, 2017). It is documented in many literature that health insurance premium continues to pose a serious financial challenge to low-income families who do not qualify for Medicare or Medicaid. The cost sharing reduction was part of the law put in place during Obama Administration. It was through legislated Patient Protection and Affordable Care Act (or ACA) of March 2010. The CSR was an amendment in ACA through the Health and Education Reconciliation Act (Rosenbaum, 2011). Many states such as Iowa embraced the CSR opportunity and used it to expand Medicaid to reach more families and adults at the low economic ladder (Saloner, et al., 2014). The CRS brought some relief in copayments and incentives to those contemplating to enroll in the various government and private health insurance marketplace.

A good healthcare policy should increase the number of Americans with healthcare insurance and eventually an access to preventive healthcare services. To the contrary, the rate of adult Americans without insurance increased by 0.4%. In the last two quarters of 2016, 10.9% of Americans adults did not have health insurance coverage. Although this rate is high compared to other developed countries it was seen as far better than the rate of uninsured US adults in 2013 (Weiner, Marks & Pauly, 2017). With the negative campaign against the ACA and the push to cut part of Medicare and Medicaid funding, more Americans were without health insurance coverage in 2017. Looking back at the trend, and according to Auter (2017), a *Gallup Poll* in the first and second quarters of 2017 shows that the rate of uninsured adult Americans rose to 11.7% from11.3%. That means there were more Americans without insurance coverage even up to going into 2018. The decline is attributed to decrease in public health insurance coverage (Berchick, Barnett &Upton, 2019).

The policy to defund coverage for the uninsured in one way or the other increases the rate of morbidity among some elderly Americans. The general public especially among the lower socioeconomic communities are also most likely to be effected. Often, these policy changes are induced by interest groups who found one way or the order to benefit from government defunding benefits for the common man. For example, a recent study found that there was no significant difference between the complications in patients who went through spinal surgery in hospitals compared to controlled population. Yet the Centers for Medicare and Medicaid Services (CMS) discontinued reimbursements for certain ill patient complications in October 2008 citing hospitals-acquired complications (HAC) (Lamsam et al, 2019).

Some people who oppose *Obamacare* did so for two main reasons.

One of the reasons was that it was unconstitutional hence people felt that they were forced to purchase health insurance or face a tax penalty (Blake, 2012). The second reason was that some parents and younger adults objected that they (the younger adults) should not be mandated to carry health insurance coverage. They quarried the need to have health insurance coverage with false assumption that young adults are not vulnerable to diseases and as such do not need healthcare services. The ACA provided the opportunity that allows young adults to stay on their family or parent(s)' health insurance plan until age 26. Despite some of these objections, the *Affordable Care Act* provided some great comfort to many Americans. This is because it provided a turning point and a new beginning to those that were left unprotected due to denial of access to healthcare services. According to a report on *Oral Health in America* by former Surgeon General, David Satcher, ACA also meant and provided an opportunity for oral health and new standard of care. Now Americans both adults and children can have access to healthcare including dental care and oral hygiene.

Unlike before more or up to 50 million people were without access to healthcare which is unacceptable (Satcher & Nottingham, 2017). This amounts to a good public health policy either directly or indirectly to benefit especially the less privileged population in the socioeconomic ladder.

Chapter Three Reference:

1. Auter, Z. (2017). Healthcare U.S. Uninsured Rate Rises to 11.7% - Gallup Poll. Retrieved from: News.gallup.com.
2. Berchick ER, Barnett JC, Upton RD. Health Insurance Coverage in the United States: 2018. Current Population Reports, P60-267(RV). U.S. Government Printing Office (Washington, DC) 2019.
3. Blake, V. (2012). The Constitutionality of the Affordable Care Act: An Update. AMA Journal of Ethics: Illuminating the

Art of Medicine. Health Law, Nov. 2012. Virtual Mentor. 2012;14(11):873-876. doi: 10.1001/virtualmentor.2012.14.11. hlaw1-1211.

4. Centers for Medicare & Medicaid Services (MMS), (2020). At Risk: Pre-Existing Conditions Could Affect 1 in 2 Americans. Centers for Medicare & Medicaid Services, April 15, 2020. Retrieved from: https://www.cms.gov/CCIIO/Resources/Forms-Reports-and-Other-Resources/preexisting.

5. Cohn, J. (2020). The ACA Repeal and The Politics of Backlash. Health Affairs. March 6, 2020. Retrieved from: https://www.healthaffairs.org/do/10.1377/hblog20200305.771008/full/.

6. Health and Human Services.gov, (2017). Coverage for pre-existing conditions: Health benefits & coverage. Health and Human Services, Assistant Secretary for Public Affairs (ASPA) January 31, 2017. Retrieved from: https://www.hhs.gov/healthcare/about-the-aca/pre-existing-conditions/index.html.

7. NCSL, 2017. (http://www.ncsl.org/programs/health/Genetics/prt.htm).

8. Webb, B.C. (2017). Breaking Down Trump's Health Care Executive Order and the End of CSR Payments. Viewpoints– UVA Public Health Science, Monday, Oct. 9th – Friday, Oct. 13th 2017.

9. Dresser, M. (1997). Healthcare Policies and Laws Medicaid Maryland General Assembly. The Baltimore Sun, November 13, 1997.

10. Solaner, et al., (2014). Pinching the Poor? Medicaid Cost Sharing Under the ACA. OBSTETRICS: Ethics, Medical Issues, and Public Policy. Obstetrical & Gynecological Survey: July 2014 - Volume 69 - Issue 7- p 384-386 doi: 10.1097/01.ogx.0000452699.74427.fc *(Saloner, Brendan; Sabik, Lindsay; Sommers, Benjamin D)*.

11. Gakh, M.; Vernick, J.S. and Rutkow, L. 2013). Public Health Report. 2013 Mar-Apr; 128(2): 127–130. PMCID: PMC3560871.

12. Layton, L., et. al. (2019). Impact of Centers for Medicare and Medicaid Services Non-Reimbursement on Hospital-Acquired Conditions Following Spine Procedures. Neurosurgery, Volume 66, Issue Supplement_1, September 2019, nyz310_106, Retrieved from: https://doi.org/10.1093/neuros/nyz310_106 Published: 20 August 2019.

13. Satcher, D. & Nottingham, J.C. (2017). Revisiting Oral Health in America. Am J Public Health. 2017 June; 107(Suppl 1): S32–S33. Published online 2017 June. doi: 10.2105/AJPH.2017.303687' PMCID: PMC5497876, PMID: 28661821. Retrieved from: https://www.ncbi.nlm.nih.gov/pmc/articles/PMC5497876/.

14. Rosenbaum, S. (2011). The Patient Protection and Affordable Care Act: Implications for Public Health Policy and Practice. Public Health Rep. 2011 Jan-Feb; 126(1): 130–135. doi: 10.1177/003335491112600118. PMCID: PMC3001814. MID: 21337939

15. Weiner, J., Marks, C., & Pauly, M., (2017). Effects of the ACA on Health Care Cost Containment. Leonard Davis Institute of Health Economics. March 2, 2017. Retrieved from: https://ldi.upenn.edu/brief/effects-aca-health-care-cost-containment.

CHAPTER 4

Public Health Implications of Bad Public Policy

General View

This chapter will discuss some implications of public policy that has not been favourable to the common people in public health view. A public health approach to public policy look for policies that are geared to protect the health of the community as a whole. The Center for Disease Control (CDC) and prevention define public health as a concept through which problems that will affect the life of individuals or any certain population is tackled as to prevent such problems. In other words a public health effort should attempt to prevent problems from happening or recurring through implementing educational programs, recommending policies and administering services to mitigate the harms.

There are different factors that make people or a group of population unhappy as against being happy. One of such driving factors is the inequalities in the society. These range from joblessness, low income earning to pressure from high premium on health and automobile insurance coverage imposed on non-affluent communities.

From all sense for equality one would think that people on the lower cadre of economic status should pay less for their smaller benefits. Why would a financially struggling individual find it difficult to obtain affordable and low insurance premium? There is a trending slogan that goes as "pay more and enjoy less" because many single family homes' taxes in low income neighbourhood are high relative to the amenities and recreational infrastructures in those communities. These pressures create daily, weekly or monthly financial burden that adds difficult life and unhappy mood. The cooperate world and some in the government seem to care less as long as the pressure is on and backed by bad public policies. Such burden manifested in terms of healthcare coverage during the early period of the pandemic. Good a thing that the US government stepped in and also took up a big role in funding COVID19 vaccine production, distribution and vaccination.

Stress of Bad Public Policy

Unhappy population is more susceptible to illnesses. One can see why the mortality rate of Corona Virus Disease 2019 (COVID19) was higher among African American communities in the United States than their Caucasian counterparts. It can be debatable that people who can reach their basic life needs with ease feel less stressed. Unlike people who cannot attain their basic life needs with ease, such group of people have to go through stressful conditions before attaining their individual needs. Other social and environmental determinants directly or indirectly caused by public policies contribute to cumulative negative outcomes. This is why many public health experts are scrambling to know why the rate of COVID19 death rate is higher in one particular race than others. Some of these socio environmental factors are listed in the CDC report on "COVID-19 Racial and Ethnic Minority Groups" (CDC, 2020). A hard look into this report implicates the need for a better public health approach to illness. It also show that medicine must focus on the health of the community as a whole. Public health is community health which implies that healthcare is vital to everyone in the society or community at all times.

Health disparities in the United States is recorded to have existed even before the modern healthcare system. Public health professionals has long advocated to limit health disparities but their efforts encounter public policies that hinder the progress. The obstacles range from calls to relocating poor communities with close proximity and exposure to chemical and stationary source chemical pollutants to paying substantial compensations to the victims. Many studies have documented findings implicating environmental injustice whereby race and low income level presented disproportionate burdens on minorities. That means their exposure to chemical pollutants and other hazardous material processing sites (Maantay, 2020). A large part of public health is promoting healthcare equity, quality and accessibility among and within every community. Socioeconomic factors also play a role in determining health equity in terms of job and labor market share. According to US Bureau of Labor Statistics Report 1082, African Americans are second to American Indians and Alaska Natives in low percentage of labor market. These group of people also have high unemployment rate (US Bureau of Labor Statistics, 2019). The less a group of population is in the labor market, the higher the social ills and health disparity. Being in the labor market is one thing and getting the fringe benefits is another. The less the skilled labor, the less the benefits such as paid family and medical leaves. Studies with data show that there is a strong racial and ethnic disparities in access to these benefits (Bartel, et al, 2019).

Universal Health Insurance Coverage (UHIC) Issue

During the William J. Clinton (the 42nd President of the United States) white House administration in (1993-2001), the issue of universal health insurance coverage (UHIC) for all Americans was a very controversial public health issue in his first term in office. The impact of costly health insurance coverage was vivid in poor inner city communities. Most members of these population have no jobs and cannot afford health insurance for themselves and their families. The fact is that during the Clinton administration, the then First Lady, Hillary Rodham-Clinton introduced and headed this policy change. It polarized the political divide in the United States Congress. This policy issue was one of the irritating factors hated by the Republican (GOP) wing of the House during the 104th Congress. The GOP revolted against the idea calling it "Big Government" that resulted in a temporary shutdown of the government.

Greater on the opposition to the proposed UHIC, were many stakeholders that played big roles in making this public health policy very controversial. The Republican Party, insurance companies, most wealthy Americans and other interest groups opted against it and still hold the same stand up till today. The Democrats on the other hand are in supports of such policy. The Democrats contend that universal health insurance coverage will serve Americans better because there is a huge health care disparity between the poor and the rich.

In the post Clinton administration presidential Contention, UHIC emerged again as a domestic policy issue. This was during the campaign platforms between President George Bush and Democratic contender, John Kerry. The UHIC public health issue was not going away in the political spectrum until those concerned about the health affair of the common Americans are satisfied. America Health Association (AHA) News opted to publish related issues as many employers started shifting rising health benefits cost to workers. The decision to publish the report is in line with the organization's mission statement and values. The Forum examined community approaches to reducing health disparities. In collaboration, many hospital leaders strove to improve health care system for patients and caregivers ("www.ahanews.com, n.d"). The idea was that universal health insurance coverage would serve these communities better but what happened at the end?

Proponents of UHIC proposed a single national health insurance system for every citizen. One would think since this was regarded as"big government control"issue, then state-based plans should have been adopted. In that case an alternate provision similar to a universal, comprehensive coverage for all inevitable hospital and health provider services should have been created (Rakich, Longest & Darr, 1992). Moreover, health insurance coverage should be publicly funded through tax payers withholding. That is, a coverage geared as a universal, comprehensive, portable between jobs and states of residence. Experts say that it can be administered publicly and be accessible without any denial due to cost. The coverage should have been designed not to incur any threats to the safety net in health care provision and services. Dental care for the elderly especially those that cannot afford the insurance coverage is a big problem also. This is because the current Medicare and Medicaid coverage in the United States experience problems with increased cost-consciousness among private providers. The ultimate victim became the patient especially the poor and elderly (Ormand et al, 1999) yet the United States spend more on healthcare of its gross domestic product (GDP) than the European countries with UHIC (McDounough et al, 1999).

Repealing and Replacing Affordable Care Act

A public policy in current healthcare coverage is a system that seem to intentionally and grossly neglect the common people. These people are left vulnerable and unprotected in terms of illness, diseases and ultimately death. Public policy is very dynamic and many regulations change with new governance. What is most important is that some policies put in place to help and protect the citizens such as in healthcare should not be revoked. As the second term of president Obama administration was coming to an end, the threat to undo *(repeal and replace)* the ACA loomed by the incoming administration. Immediately after the 45th president was sworn in on January 20, 2017 the bell to repeal and replace Obamacare rang louder and louder. On May 4, 2017, the House Republican party as the majority in the house passed a bill to repeal and replace the American Affordable Healthcare Act, (Obamacare).

How elected officials care for protecting the common American is a concern when it comes to certain public policy. One may ask, do the elected officials really care when it comes down to choosing between their personal interests, expected value and anticipated rewards versus protecting the common man? This book is not focused to be critical of the elected officials rather to examine few points why it views certain public policy particularly those related to public health has failed to protect the people on the lower economic ladder. For example, since after the symbolic repeal of the ACA, attempts to get the Senate to pass the bill to replace it with the new proposed America Health Care (AHA) has met obstacles. On June 27, 2017 the Senate failed for the third time to muster enough vote to pass the GOP House Bill to replace the *Obamacare*. Some of the reasons behind the insufficient votes to move the bill forwards include the elimination of the restrictions on health insurance organizations.

Under ACA, insurance companies as supposed to be non-for profit entities were required to invest back 85% of their revenues into the system which would lower the health coverage cost. That means they are allowed to benefit on 15-20% of the profit made. Another reason is the funding cut in Medicare and Medicaid at many state levels (Barlas, 2012). Although the cuts and reductions in Medicare and Medicaid funding look ludicrous to some people and the potential victims but the law-makers see it as a way of compromise in both chambers in order to avoid unnecessary impasses in running the government at both federal and some state governments. It is also viewed as one of the cracks through which the government can reduce budget deficits (Butler, 2018). Despite these rationales for cutting Medicare and Medicaid funding, the prime concern in public health perspective is whether there is a hidden motive in making these cuts and the impact it have on those affected (HCUP, 2009). Moreover, on 25Th June 2020 President Trump administration filed a legal brief to the United Stated Supreme Court asking the court to annul the Affordable Care Act (The Wall Street Journal, 2020).

Should the Supreme Court uphold the request, it will be a difficult condition for many Americans who cannot afford out-of-pocket medical expenses. According to Caldwell (2017) majority of Americans showed great dissatisfaction with the 115th US congress led by Republican majority. This was the reason three Republican senators, John McCain (now late), Susan Collins and Lisa Murkowski voted with all Democrats against the bill to repeal Obamacare (KFF, 2021). The point to make here is that a good public health policy that benefits the average citizen is always welcomed by the majority of the citizens. On the other hand public policy that is motivated for the advantage of a few becomes very controversial and less supported by the mass. Several pools showed that more than 51% of Americans oppose the senate bill of the insurance law to repeal and replace the ACA or Obamacare.

The prosed bill will hurt many Americans and some states are not happy with the intension to shift the bigger responsibilities of healthcare to the states. For instance, in the state of Tennessee, more people rely on Medicare and Medicaid (KFF, 2017) and cutting funding of the program will leave many of its residents without access to healthcare services. Although there are other sections of the ACA that were unpopular among many Americans, this has been due to improper understanding of the law. Moreover, there has also been overblown and polarized deceptive advertisements and negative health policy messages by opponents of the law. The irony of the ACA among many adult Americans who dearly need the Affordable Care Act is the negative policy communication. The law has been presented in biased policy language as *Obamacare*. This became a turnoff to many middle-class at the edge and low income American to reject the ACA without the knowledge that the Affordable Care Act is the same health policy as the *Obamacare*. Now that the republican House and Senate bill respectively has the potential to increase the number of uninsured Americans, people are now calling to reject the repeal of *Obamacare*.

The proposed bills will defund many entitlement programs that protect many low income people from going uninsured. The reasons for defunding certain government programs include a measure to reduce federal deficit and shrink government overreach on social programs. There is also a theory that it is a means of maybe, to indirectly force people out from government dependency. More so, there could be other reasons that make sense only to the proponents of the bill. According to Planned Parenthood, the proposed bill is *drafted in secret and that majority of Americans reject such disregard to the common people with intension to block millions of patients from care by "defunding"* its organization (Planned Parenthood, n.d). In the state of Nevada for instance some organized groups including the Planned Parenthood are calling people to reach their senators to demand a *No to Trumpcare* ("Call Your Senator," n.d.). Analysis by the Congressional Budget Office (CBO) revealed that the amendment provided in the Senate health bill will make it difficult for many Americans to be able to purchase health insurance coverage. The estimate indicated that about 22 million more Americans will become uninsured (Park, 2017). This is a gross negative implication of bad public policy that affect public health.

Chapter Four References

1. America Health Association, (n.d). Hospital Leaders Strove to Improve Healthcare System for Patients and Caregivers. Retrieved from: www.ahanews.com.
2. Barlas, S. (2012). State Cutbacks to Medicaid May Hit Hospitals Hard: *New Federal Reductions Might Compound the Stress*. Journal of Pharmacy & Therapeutics v.37(10); 2012 Oct PMC3474445. MediMedia USA, Inc.

3. Bartle AP, Kim S, Nam J, Rossin-Slater M, Ruhm C, Waldfogel J. Racial and ethnic disparities in access to and use of paid family and medical leave: evidence from four nationally representative datasets, Monthly Labor Review, U.S. Bureau of Labor Statistics, January 2019. https://doi.org/10.21916/mlr.2019.2.

4. Butler, M.S. (2018). Don't Let Budget Cuts Wreck Medicare Reform. JAMA. 2018;319(10):970-971. doi:10.1001/jama.2018.1439

5. Caldwell, L. A. (2017). Obamacare stays. For now. NBC News. July 28, 2017.

6. CDC, (2020). COVID-19 Racial and Ethnic Minority Groups. Retrieved from: www.ahanews.com.

7. Healthcare Cost and Utilization Project (HCUP): Nationwide Emergency Department Sample (NEDS) HCUP, Rockville, MD: Agency for Healthcare Research and Quality; 2009. Retrieved from: https://www.hcup-us.ahrq.gov/nedsoverview.jsp.

8. Healthcare Cost and Utilization Project (HCUP): Nationwide Emergency Department Sample (NEDS), HCUP, Rockville, MD: Agency for Healthcare Research and Quality; 2009. Retrieved from: https://www.hcup-us.ahrq.gov/nedsoverview.jsp.

9. Kaiser Family Foundation (KFF), (2017). Medicaid's Role in Tennessee: AP Investigate the State of the Nation's Public Health Infrastructure. KFF's Kaiser Health News (KHN), Jul 21, 2017.

10. KFF (Kaiser Family Foundation), (2021). KFF Health Tracking Poll: The Public's Views on the ACA Published: Mar 03, 2021.

11. Maantay, J. (2002). Mapping Environmental Injustices: Pitfalls and Potential of GeographicInformation Systems in Assessing Environmental Health and Equity. Department of Geology and Geography, Lehman College, City University of

New York, Bronx, New York, USA. Environmental Health Perspectives • VOLUME 110 | SUPPLEMENT 2 | April 2002.

12. McDounough, J. E. et al, (1999). Healthcare policy: The basics: http://www.accessproject.org/downloads/the-basics.pdf. Website retrieved June 7, 2020.

13. Ormand, B. et al (1999). Health care for the low-income people in the District of Columbia.http://www,urban.org.health/dc_lowincome.html. Website retrieved August 15, 2020.

14. Park, E., (2017). New CBO Estimate: Still 22 Million More Uninsured Under Revised Senate Republican Health Bill. https://www.cbpp.org/research/health/new-cbo-estimate-still-22-million-more-uninsured-under-revised-senate-republican.

15. Planned Parenthood, (n.d.). Call Your Senators to demand a *No to Trumpcare*. Retrieved March January 25, 2020 from: https://www.istandwithpp.org/call.

16. Rakich, J. S., Longest, Jr, B.B, & Darr, K., (1992). Managing health services organization (3rd edition). Health Profession Press, London; p78-88.

17. US Bureau of Labor Statistics, (2018). Report 1082, Labor force characteristics by race and ethnicity, 2018. October 2019. https://www.bls.gov/opub/reports/race-and-eth List: 2/18/2021.

18. Wall Street Journal, (2020). Trump Administration Asks Supreme Court to Invalidate Affordable Care Act. The Wall Street Journal, June 30 (2020).

CHAPTER 5

Evidence-Based Facts and Epidemiology of Lead Poisoning

The Effect On A Population Health

The research and practice community surmised that blood lead screenings to identify and treat children for elevated blood lead levels reduces the risk of childhood lead poisoning. This is important particularly in low-income urban communities (Bloch, Guthrine, & Rosenblum, 2000). However, it was not clear what the ultimate benefits, expectations, values, and implications of the disclosure policy were. In public policy formation and models, decisions are often influenced by a variety of factors. These include predictions, policy choice and interest groups (Porter & Hicks, 1999). Other influencing factors comprise effectiveness of alternate options, cost-benefit analysis, values and motives (Matanoski, 2001). It has also been documented that there is a correlation between socioeconomic status and prevalence of lead-based paint exposure in the urban communities. Households in the lower economic ladder tend to occupy homes built before 1950. These homes have lead-based paint finished walls, ceilings and doors. These include homes in the urban and rural areas (Kegler, & Malcoe, 2004), (LACPH, 2006).

As these homes aged into the 1970s and beyond, the building structures of these homes began to weather. The resultant impact is shading off lead coated paint chips and dust in both the interior and exteriors surfaces. Families with toddlers in such homes could have started noticing their crawling kids pick and ingesting lead-based paint chips. It is not uncommon that little children pick up tiny objects and put into their mouth as they crawl around the house unless they are strictly and effectively watched. It is through such scenario that a child accumulate loads of lead dust and chips by ingesting or inhaling up to unhealthy concentration up to $10\mu g/dL$. In many cases the lead dust load become too high in their blood stream (Agency for Toxic Substances and Disease Registry [ATSDR], 1997).

With increased medical manifestation of lead-based paint exposure, the epidemiology of lead poisoning in the United States became a formidable population health issue not to be neglected. The Centers for Disease Control and Prevention (CDC) as a vital organ for the United States Department of Health and Human Services incorporated funding, health promotion programs and research to investigate, analyze and advice on how to mitigate the problem of lead-based paint poisoning of children. This move was no less than CDC's action on other prevailing diseases that cause morbidity and mortality among human population. That meant taking lead poisoning like any other such as emerging infectious diseases, food and waterborne diseases, respiratory infections, birth defects or obesity (Siegel, & Doner, 2004).

As a track in public health field, epidemiological studies on childhood lead-based paint poisoning provided evidence of an association between exposure to lead-based paint with older homes built in mid-twentieth (20th) century in the United States (CDC, 1997). Markowitz (2000) expressed that evidence of morbidity and poisoning resulting from exposure to lead-based paint was not lacking among children leaving in older homes in low income urban communities. Chung, Webb, Clampet-Lundquist, and Campbell (2001) documented that some of the negative outcomes of lead-based paint exposure include slow developments in intelligence, decreased cognitive ability, impaired neurobehavioral development, diminished stature, hearing abnormalities and learning problems. Other effects include an increase in tooth decays (Matte, 1999). Stroop, Dietrich, Hunt, Suddendorf, and Giangiacomo (2000) implicated fetal lead encephalopathy among unborn babies of mothers living in homes with a high risk of lead-based paint or who were exposed to lead paint dust during pregnancy.

Often, policy makers neglect scientific data generated for evidenced-based policy decisions. This happens because groups who lobby to ensure that their own interests are protected have influenced the policy makers' objective reasoning (Greenberg, 1992). Sommer (2001) argued that effective public health policy undergoes a process, and factors such as politics, interest groups, public opinion polls, the media, new technology, evidence, data, and the economic cost of a health intervention program can influence public health policy. As these factors become real, Sommer asked, "how else can it be explained that our [United States] ban on lead paint came over half a century after Australia's?" (Summer, 2001). The obvious answer is that values, motives and interests played a major role and may have influenced the delay. These are the attributes of the expectancy value theory.

Evidence-Based Facts

It is worthy to note that the effectiveness of a public health program is determined by process, impact and outcome evaluations of the program. Moreover, implementation and meeting the goal for which the program is designed must be on the focus. This is a concept that transcends to application of evidenced-based policy and practice in public health service delivery. Evidence-based concept should be employed to utilize the maximum resource to better the health of the population of the society. The public health agencies and services sector is the primary body with the duty to protect and promote the population's health and well-being. A typical example of the opposite is the pediatric environmental problem relative to elevated blood lead levels in children in Flint, Michigan due to contaminated drinking water (Hanna-Attisha et al, 2016). This crisis was associated with the failure of the city public works department and other appropriate authorities in protecting the citizens from the risk of consuming bad quality drinking water. It is also the primary responsibility of the public health agencies to endorse and implement policies and practice that are of uttermost benefit to the citizens and their communities. This include public school buildings and its environs. It is obvious that school-aged children spend part of their time five days a week during in-class learnings sessions. As part of pediatric environmental health, local institutions should also play roles to be heard in solving critical pediatric environmental health problems (Etzel & Balk, 2011). It is ironic to allow social factors to undermine the need to eradicate lead poisoning of children in any society (Boseila, Gabr & Hakim, 2004) and with appropriate programs (Zierold & Anderson, 2004).

The application of evidenced-based policy and practice concept should be utilized in public health service and delivery. The practice should encompass the best available evidence from wide range of sources for decision making in public health. The application should be analogous to that of "the Best Available Technology (BET) as in industries environmental pollution control. There is a need for evidence-based policy and practice to provide and deliver the appropriate health services to the society and community. Based on various references, the United States have the best technology in health equipment and practice, and also spend more on health, yet there is a huge health disparity in the USA compared to other industrialized nations (McDounough, et al, 1999), (Rakisc & Longest, 1992).

On this frame of reference, one could ask, what is the role of scientific analysis in health policy formation? Some schools of thought contend that science and scientific analysis are complementary to each other and are philosophical (Rosenberg, 2000) requiring critical thinking in application and utilization. Based on this framework the role of scientific analysis in health policy formation is very important as it enlightens and explain on what can be done, modified, optimized and utilized for a better health services delivery for the general population. Technical expertise is a product of scientific research and analysis. It is also an indicative of proper direction as it prescribes for policy formation in a direct or indirect call to the policy makers. In health policy, these prescriptions by scientific findings and analysis do not directly always yield into practical policy formation. Rather, in a given policy stage they do play roles as tools for advocates, interest groups and bureaucrats. It also enable other forces or stakeholders in the course of finding a solution for appropriate health policies.

One such example is the sequencing of the human genome announced in 2000. Evidenced based data revealed that through this scientific discovery, medical information and predictive genetic testing enabled researchers to identify risk for many common human diseases. It has also been acknowledged as a means that can help reduce or correct genetic profiling (Drenkard & Ferguson, 2002). Analysis of this scientific breakthrough has created various schools of thought. Those against genetic profiling contend that it will cause increase in discrimination in employment, education, healthcare and insurance. Others advocate for a voluntary and consent based genetic testing (Drenkard & Ferguson, 2002). In the United States, many states have Genetic Privacy Laws (GPL) for the use of genetic testing and profiling. GPL is recommended and provided by the National Conference of State Legislatures (NCSL) (Johnson, 2007). Another role of scientific analysis in health policy is the use of the analysis and evidence for health services strategies in health management agenda in areas of intervention and other clinical decision making. For example, procedures, and practices that does more harm than good be stopped or slowed and vice versa (Muir-Gray, 2001).

In reviewing policies that shaped the impact of lead exposure experiences in urban communities, LeBrón et al. (2019) expressed that many policies on lead exposure were rather aimed to moderating the impact of exposure than prevention of exposure. It also became implicit that lead policies largely focused on establishing hazardous lead exposure levels in settings consumer products, disclosing lead hazards, and remediating lead paint. It also put more emphasis on mitigating exposures once children have been exposed to lead (as indicated by elevated child blood lead levels), rather than prevention. As noted by many concerned organizations and groups, prevention of childhood lead poisoning should have been a priority for lead-based paint hazard policy (AAPCEH, 2016). Some clauses in the policy provided evidence that there are gaps in existing policies as to provoke specific recommendations to prevent lead exposures and to promote health equity (Iregbu, 2008).

As indicated in Iregbu (2008), identifying a program to eliminate childhood lead poisoning has been a concern of the public health agencies in the United States since the early 1970s. A socioeconomic implication of childhood lead poisoning revealed that 21.9% of childhood lead poisoning was among poor black children with families living in houses built prior 1946. Their blood lead levels (BLLs) was > 10ug/dL (CDC, 1997). Though this level is widely agreed to be the clinical level for adverse effect but i*n public health perspective there is no blood lead level in children considered as safe.* This concept has triggered some question on what is the appropriate level or legal limit of childhood lead exposure (Bernard, 2003). The reason is that irrespective of the blood level, whether really low or just below EBLL it has been documented that such victims (children) may suffer encephalopathy (Holstege, Rowden & Griesemer, 2006). They may also exhibit impaired IQ, inability to pay attention in class and a tendency of low academic achievement (NCEH, 2019). The presence of lead-based paint dust and chips posing a risk to a specific population has been a problem that pediatricians would fault policy makers (AAP, 2020), (Lanphear, Eberly & Howard, 2000). As frontline workers in observing the victims, they play the crucial role in preventing childhood lead exposure even at providing guidelines on how to diagnose the illness (Miller, 2011). They also recommend treatment options for lead poisoning in children, and further advocate for public health measures to address the problem (AAP, 2020). Many advocates for environmental justice (Evans & Marcynyszyn, 2004) and safer homes fault housing policies (Brown et al., 2001). They encouraged encouraged intensive lead exposure screening for targeted communities (Dignam et al., 2004) as a measure to reduce childhood lead poisoning.

Chapter Five Reference

1. Agency for Toxic Substances and Disease Registry (ATSDR). (1997). Lead and your health. ATSDR, August, 1997.

2. American Academy of Pediatrics (AAP), (2020). Lead Exposure and Lead Poisoning. American Academy of Pediatrics; Professional Resources 2020. Retrieved August 26, 2020 from: https://www.aap.org/en-us/advocacy-and-policy/aap-health-initiatives/lead-exposure/Pages/default.aspx.

3. American Academy of Pediatrics Council on Environmental Health (AAPCEH), (2016). Prevention of childhood lead toxicity. Pediatrics: 2016 138(1). Epub 2016 Jun20; Pediatrics. Retrieved May 28, 2020 from: http://dx.doi.org/10.1542/peds.2016-1493. [PubMed].

4. Bernard, S. M. (2003). Should the Centers for Disease Control and Prevention's childhood lead poisoning intervention level be lowered? American Journal of Public Health, 93 (8), 1253-1264.

5. Bloch, A. B., Guthrine, A. M., & Rosenblum, L. R. (2000). Recommendations for blood lead levels screening of young children enrolled in Medicaid: Targeting a group at high risk. *Mortality and Morbidity Weekly Report*, *49* (14), 391-422.

6. Boseila, S. A., Gabr, G. A., & Hakim, I. A. (2004). Blood lead level in Egyptian children: Influence of social and environmental factors. *American Journal of Public Health, 94* (1), 44-48.

7. Brown, M. J., Gardner, J., Sargent, J. D., Swartz, K., Hu, H., & Timperi, R. (2001). The effectiveness of housing policies in reducing children's lead exposure. The American Journal of Public Health, 91(4), 621-624.

8. CDC, (1997). Screening young children for lead poisoning: Guidance for state and local public health officials (pp. 13-20). CDC, Atlanta, GA. Nov. 1997.

9. Chung, E. K., Webb, D., Clampet-Lundquist, S and Campbell, C. (2001). A comparison of elevated blood lead levels among children living in foster care, their siblings, and the general population. Pediatric 107(5). Retrieved from http://www.pediatrics.aapublications.org.

10. Dignam, T. A., Evens, A., Eduard, E., Ramirez, S. Caldwell, K. L., & Kilpatrick, N., et al. (2004). High-intensity targeted screening for elevated blood lead levels among children in two inner-city Chicago communities. *American Journal of Public Health, 94* (11), 1951-1945.

11. Drenkard, K and Ferguson, S., (2002). Genetic testing and discrimination – From research to policy in paediatric nursing: Case example – Virginia.

12. Etzel, R.A., Balk. S.J. (2018). Pediatric environmental health, 4th Edition: American Academy of Pediatrics Council of Environmental Health. American Academy of Pediatrics, December 1, 2018.

13. Evans, G. W., & Marcynyszyn, L. A. (2004). Environmental justice, cummulative environmrntal risk, and health among low- and middle-income children in upstate New York. American Journal of Public Health, 94 (11), 1942-1948.

14. Greenberg, M. (1992). Impediments to basing government health policies on science in the United States. *Social Science & Medicine, 35* (4), 531-540.

15. Hanna-Attisha M., LaChance J., Sadler R.C., Schnepp A.C.(2026). Elevated blood lead levels in children associated with the flint drinking water crisis: A spatial analysis of risk and public health response. Am. J. Public Health. 2016;106:283–290. doi: 10.2105/AJPH.2015.303003.

16. Holstege, C. P., Rowden, A. K., & Griesemer, D. (2006). Lead encephalopathy. *eMedicine*. Retrieved from http://www. emedicine.com

17. Iregbu, C. A., (2008). Lead Paint Disclosure Policy: Implications for Eliminating Childhood Lead Exposure in Baltimore City, 2008, University of Michigan Publishers. Also: Barnes and Noble Published online July 2011.

18. Johnson, A. (2007). Plunging Into the Gene Pool. State Genetics Legislation Database of 2004-2007, March 2007. Retrieved from July 24, 2020 from: www.ncsl.org/programs/ health/Genetics/prt.htm).

19. Kegler, M. C., & Malcoe, H. L. (2004). Results from a lay health advisor intervention to prevent lead poisoning among rural Native American children. *American Journal of Public Health, 94* (10), 1730-1735.

20. Lanphear, B. P, Eberly, S., & Howard, C. R. (2000). Long-term effect of dust control on blood lead concentrations. *Pediatrics, 106* (4), 820-829.

21. LeBrón et al., (2019). The State of Public Health Lead Policies: Implications for Urban Health Inequities and Recommendations for Health Equity. Int J Environ Res Public Health. 2019 Mar; 16(6): 1064. Published online 2019 Mar 24. doi: 10.3390/ijerph16061064 PMCID: PMC6466291 PMID: 30909658.

22. Los Angeles County Public Health (LACPH), (2006). Lead report: Census/surveillance. LACPH June 2006. Retrieved from http://ww.lapublichealth.org.

23. Markowitz, M. (2000). Lead poisoning. Pediatric Review, 21 (1), 327-335.

24. Matanoski, G., (2001). Conflicts between two cultures: Implications for epidemiologic researchers in communicating with policy-makers. American Journal of Epidemiology, Vol.154, No.12, S36-S42.

25. Matte, T. D. (1999). Reducing blood lead levels: Benefits and strategies. Journal of the American Medical Association, 281 (24), 2340-2348.

26. McDounough, J. E. et al, (1999). Healthcare policy: The basics http://www.accessproject.org/downloads/the-basics.pdf. Website retrieved June 7, 2005.

27. Muir Gray, J.A, (2001). Evidenced-based healthcare: How to make health policy and management decisions (2nd ed) Edinburg: Churchill Livingstone, p37-62.

28. National Center for Environmental Health (NCEH), (2019). Lead Poisoning Prevention. NCEH; Division of Environmental Health Science and Practice. July 30, 2019.

29. Porter, R, W., & Hicks, I. (1999). Knowledge utilization and the process of policy formation. Retrieved from http//sara.aed.org.

30. Siegel, M., & Doner, L. (2004). Marketing public health: Strategies to promote social change. Boston, MA: Jones and Bartlett.

31. Sommer, A. (2001). How public health policy is created: Scientific process and political reality. *American Journal of Epidemiology, 154* (12), S4-S6.

32. Stroop, D. M., Dietrich, K. N., Hunt, A. N., Suddendorf, L. R., and Giangiacomo, M. (2000). Lead-based paint health risk assessment in dependent children living in military housing. *Public Health Reports, 117* (5), 446-452.

33. Rakich, J.S., Longest, Jr, B.B, & Darr, K., (1992). Managing health services organization (3rd edition). Health Profession Press, London; p78-88.

34. Rosenberg, A., (2000). Philosophy of science: A contemporary introduction. New York, NY: Routledge; p1-4.

35. Zierold, K. M., & Anderson, H. (2004). Trends in blood lead levels among children enrolled in the special supplemental nutrition program for women, infants, and children from 1996 to 2000. *American Journal of Public Health, 94* (9), 1513-1518.

CHAPTER 6

Lead Based Paint Public Health Issue

Baltimore City Example

This chapter will provide a review of implication of public policy relative to lead-based paint poisoning as a public health problem in the United States using Baltimore City example. Numerous books, articles and documentaries has shown that lead poisoning of children 6 years and younger was identified as one of the major public health problems in the United States in the early 1970s (Iregbu, 2008). Although childhood lead poisoning in the United States have come under control by the early 2000s, the epidemic is still chided among public health professionals and environmental justice group. The advocacy is against public health policy that neglected non-affluent urban families with the demise of childhood lead poisoning and related traits. In 2015, the death of Freddie Gray, a 25 year old African American young man who died in hospital from spinal injuries sustained during his encounter with the police, resulted in a rioting and protracted civil protest in Baltimore City. Of importance to this chapter and book is the attribute to Mr. Gray having suffered childhood lead-based paint exposure (McCoy, 2015) in Baltimore City during his childhood.

Mr. Gray lived in the Baltimore City neighborhood with older homes in the "21217" zip code area. This is a non-affluent community of Sandtown-Winchester in predictive area of high risk for lead poisoning (MDE, 1999) as indicated in figure 6.1. The neighborhood is predominantly African Americans making up 97.68% of the population as shown in Appendix-A. How this condition affected his life is out of scope of this book. However, there are numerous evidence based data that children exposed to lead do experience some health issues including early academic instability (Hauptman, Bruccoleri & Woolf, 2017). Baltimore City has many of such neighborhoods and homes (Images for Baltimore, 2006). Such shortcomings may likely affect their life during teenage and young adulthood. Policy makers could have involved communities affected by lead-based paint expose in one way or the other to integrate community actions. One such example could be encouraging better social and capacity building for interventions to improve health equity and in mitigating childhood lead poisoning. Referencing available epidemiological data in the less affluent communities (Wallerstein, Yen & Syme, 2011) would have served well for such purpose.

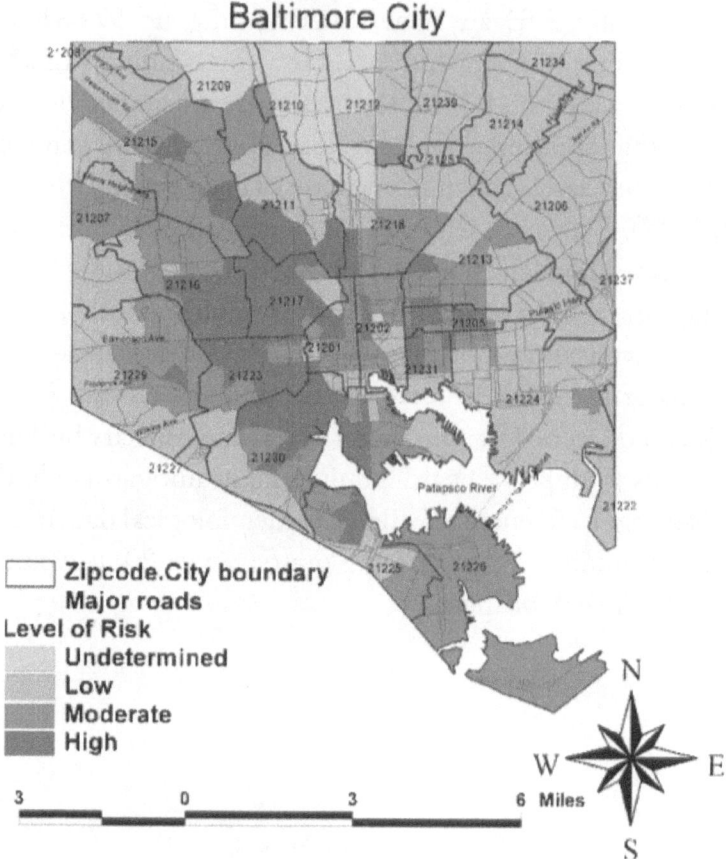

MARYLAND DEPARTMENT OF THE ENVIRONMENT
Lead Poisoning Prevention Program
Predicted Areas of Risk for Lead Poisoning by Census Tract
With Zip Code Overlay
For Children Under 6 Years of Age
Based on the Maryland Model (1999)

Baltimore City

Figure 6.1: Predicted Areas of Risk for Childhood
Lead Poisoning in Baltimore City
Source: Maryland Department of the Environment.

In a cost-benefit analysis on investments that mitigated and controlled childhood lead poisoning, Gould (2009) concluded that there was a good return on investment in controlling child lead exposure and poisoning in the United States. The awareness of lead-based paint problem in older homes generated national and public health attention in the 1970s. It was documented that approximately 890,000 American children had blood lead levels (BLLs) equal to 10μg/dL or greater (CDC, 1997). When the BLLs equal to 10μg/dL or higher it is regarded or defined as an elevated childhood blood level (EBLL). Many children with EBBLs surfer the risk of impaired learning ability (CDC, 2015). In addition, some may experience off-track behavior. About 21.9% of African American children were identified with this condition of EBLL (ATSDR, 1997) during the height of lead-based paint poisoning in the nation. In public health perspective there is no blood lead level in children considered as safe. The reason is that irrespective of the blood level whether really low or just below EBLL it has been documented that such victims (children) may suffer impaired IQ, exhibit inability to pay attention in class and tendency of low academic achievement (NCEH, 2019). In contrast, children in Alaska did not suffer from elevated blood lead levels.

The Baltimore City example is a review of a study by Iregbu (2008) in which the target Community and Population was taken from the housing units within Baltimore City's limits using available secondary data. It utilized both low-income and more affluent communities in the City. Selecting criteria for the communities in the study was based on row-houses and single-family homes built before 1950 as well as multiple dwelling rental apartments built prior to 1978. These were residential buildings completed before the lead-based paint ban in the United States. It also considered households living below the federal poverty income ratio. Utilizing the 2000 United States Census data it is obvious that African Americans have the highest population in Baltimore City with 64.9% as shown in table 6.1 below (Iregbu, 2008).

Table 6.1: Using 2000 and Updated 2005 Average Census Data on Race/Ethnic Groups to Relate Childhood Lead-Based Paint Poisoning in Baltimore

Total Population, 2000	651,154
Living in same house in1995 and 2000, pct 5 yrs old & over	57.1%
Population of persons under 5 years old	47,091
Percent of population with high school diploma, age 25+	68.4%
Percent of population with bachelor's degree or higher, age 25+	19.1%
Total number of housing units, 2005	294,262
Occupied housing units	242,978
Owner-occupied housing units	123,532
Renter-occupied housing units (2005)	119,446
Vacant housing units (2005)	51,248
Percent of vacant housing units	17.4%
Homeownership rate, 2000	50.3%
Housing units in multi-unit structures, percent in 2000	34.8%
Median value of owner-occupied housing units, 2000	$69,100
Total number of households, 2000	257,996
Average number of persons per household, 2000	2.42
Median household income, 2003	$29,066
Percent of population in labor force, age 16 year and older	63.6%
Percent of population below poverty level, 2003	19.6%
White persons' percent in 2005	*31.7%*
Black persons' percent in 2005	*64.9%*
American Indians and Alaskan Native persons' percent in 2005	*0.3%*
Asian persons' percent in 2005	*1.9%*

Hispanic or Latino Origin persons' percent in 2005	2.2%
Native Hawaiian and Other Pacific Islanders' percent in 2005	0.1%

Source: Iregbu (2008) from Baltimore City Department of Planning [BCDP], 2001 Report of US 2000 Census Data.

As this chapter try to explain how some bad public policy affect the health of the citizens, it must be acknowoleged that an illhealth of any one member in a household may have a direct or indirect impact on others in the same family circle either the young or the old. Literature and reports on the prevalence of lead-based paint poisoning in Baltimore City between January and December 1997 and according to the data obtained from Maryland Department of the Environment lead registry revealed that there were a total of one thousand two hundred thirty three (1,233) children identified as clinically lead poisoned in the state of Maryland. The troubling aspect of this finding was that children in Baltimore City alone accounted for 1,030 of the total number. Table 6.2 shows the prevalence of childhood lead poisoning in Baltimore City compared to other Maryland jurisdictions.

Table 6.2: Childhood Lead Registry Blood Lead Screening Among Children 0-72 Months (as reported to CLR for 1/1/97-12/3/97).

Counties (Co.)	#of Children below 6 yrs	Screened Number Percent	Lead Exposed Number Percent	Lead Poisoned Number Percent
Allegany	4790	1200 25.1%	72 6.0%	8 0.7%
Anne Arundel	39,471	5226 13.2%	179 3.4%	20 0.4%
Baltimore City	61,102	21,423 35.1%	5,983 27.9%	1,030 4.8%
Baltimore Co.	55,757	7,921 14.2%	427 5.4%	52 0.7%
Calvert	6,015	531 8.8%	10 1.9%	1 0.2%
Caroline	2,597	503 19.4%	56 11.1%	5 1.0%
Carroll	12,620	756 6.0%	40 5.3%	8 1.1%
Cecil	7,043	409 5.8%	22 5.4%	7 1.7%
Charles	11,195	1,124 10.0%	18 1.6%	0 0.0%
Dorchester	2,301	432 18.8%	62 14.4%	9 2.1%
Frederick	16,002	1,122 7.0%	57 5.1%	11 1.0%
Garrett	2,301	405 17.6%	6 1.5%	0 0.0%
Harford	19,437	1,466 7.5%	43 3.0%	4 0.3%
Howard	20,522	1,192 5.8%	22 1.8%	0 0.0%
Kent	1,349	281 20.8%	16 5.7%	2 0.7%
Montgomery	70,843	7,709 10.9%	112 1.5%	15 0.2%
Prince George	69,315	10,286 14.8%	200 2.0%	30 0.3%
Queen Anne	3,127	371 11.9%	17 4.5%	2 0.5%
Somerset	1,459	414 28.4%	50 12.1%	5 1.2%
St. Mary	8,551	976 11.4%	52 5.3%	4 0.4%
Talbot	2,300	371 16.1%	15 4.1%	1 0.3%
Washington	9,599	490 5.1%	26 5.3%	4 0.8%
Wicomico	6,545	868 13.3%	110 12.7%	12 1.4%
Worchester	3,098	493 15.9%	42 8.5%	2 0.4%
Unknown	000%	1,149 000%	126 000%	1 000%
Total	437,339	67,118 15.3%	7,763 11.6%	1,233 1.8%

Source. From Maryland Department of Environment-Lead Poisoning Prevention Program, Childhood Lead Surveillance in Maryland, 1997 Annual Report.

In Maryland, the childhood lead registry report for January 1,

1997 to December 31, 1997 showed that a total of 67,118 children aged 0-72 months were screened for lead-based paint exposure in 24 jurisdictions including Baltimore City. Out of this number 7,763 tested positive for lead based paint exposure. Breaking down these numbers futher from the table 6.2, it shows that 1,030 children in Baltimore City were confirmed as clinically lead poisoned out of 1,233 under same category in the entire State of Maryland. This can be attributed from the fact that the city of Baltimore accounted for the highest percentage of exposure at 27.9% based on the number screened (21, 423) and the number exposed (5,983). On converting this number to percentage it represented 4.8% of children that were lead-based paint poisoned in Baltimore City from the number of children screened during the above specific period (MED, 1998). This showed that Baltimore City had the highest childhood lead poisoining than the other twenty three (23) jurisdictions in the state of Maryland.

The Right To Know Policy

The convolutedness of *The Right To Know Policy or Disclosure Policy* is that property owners are only required to disclose all known information about lead-based paint or potential lead-based paint hazard in and around their property. As the seller of a residential building or as the property owner, such individual is obligated to disclose any lead-based paint related facts such as the actual year the house was built, condition of the painted surfaces and others (USEPA Code of Federal Registry 40, 745, 1992). Also, the policy demanded that sellers allow the homebuyer(s) a10-day period to conduct an independent lead-based paint inspection or risk assessment for lead-based paint or lead-based paint hazards (Iregbu, 2008). The US Environmental Protection Agency document (EPA-747-F-96-001 of 1996) spelled out these guidelines but the property owner is not compelled to allow such inspection process. Hence only by mutual agreement in writing to when and or if the inspection must be conducted.

Based on the above frame of reference, the potential renters or buyers can waive the inspection opportunity. If that option is taken for fear of losing the chance to rent or buy the house the renter or buyer bears the economic or other potential risk of exposure to lead-based paint. In public health perspective, this option of non-obligatory clause to bear the cost of lead-based paint inspection and abatement stood as the weakness of the policy. It is in no doubt that this policy failed to protect the low-income members of the society who try to find a shelter for the family. On the other hand the policy protected the more affluent property owners or sellers. This is because as long as the seller provided the EPA pamphlet known as *The Right To Know* and other required notifications for signature and date, the next action lies on the buyer. Once the potential occupant (buyer) of the property sign and date the agreement to move in, the property owner does not bear any fault. At this point he or she is relieved of the responsibility to perform lead-based paint abatement or risk reduction on the property (Iregbu, 2008) and (EPA & HUD, 1998).

A simple explanation of the Lead-based paint Disclosure Policy on residential homes gives a problem free scenario. Nevertheless, a hard look into the policy will find that it was prone to create a big public health calamity to a certain population. That is environmental problem for children leaving in low income urban communities. It amounted to a generation exposed to indoor environmental risk that the laws ignored (Abell Foundation, 2002). Some questions to ask include how did the policy influence lead abatements in housing units in the target populations? Whereas one can also argue whether the policy was meant for pro-abatement or against lead-based paint abatement by the property owners. If abatement substantially or completely eliminates the mass-load of lead from a home as documented by intervention research, it is better to enforce it as law than making it optional. In that way, the policy could have embedded some sort of tactical enforcement action targeting pre-1950 homes

rented, leased, or sold to low-income families in the urban and inner
cities across the nation (Iregbu, 2008). Plot in figure 6.2 show the
trend of lead-based paint abatement or other risk reduction on the
properties occupied by affluent and non-affluent home owners in
Baltimore City.

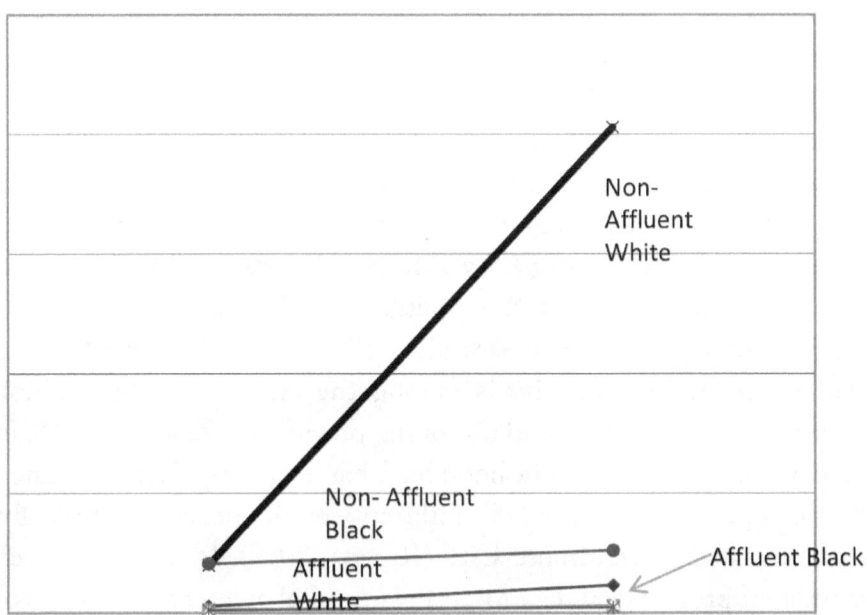

**Figure 6:2 Percent of Housing Units Receiving Lead Abatement
and Other Risk-Reduction Measures in Black, White, Affluent
and Non-Affluent Baltimore City.**
Source: Iregbu 2008.

The fact is that lead-based paint exposure and poisoning in older
homes is not an infectious disease like Human Immunodeficiency
Virus/Acquired Immune-deficiency Syndrome (HIV/AIDS) or worst
as Corona Virus of 2019 (COVID19). Hence the condition is not
transmittable from person to person by touch or contact. On the
ground of this situation childhood lead-based paint poisoning was
and is preventable. It could have been100% preventable (NCEH,

2019) on the early incidences among children in urban communities with low-income populations through good public health policy.

What The Policy Did Not Do

Bad public policy often a times are prone to some kind of unintended socioeconomic implications. The lead-based paint disclosure policy with the clause of *The Right To Know* is one of such public policy that did not help prevent childhood lead-based paint exposure and poisoning. The children of low-income families living in urban areas suffered the unintended consequence as specific population. In Baltimore City African American children make up almost one quarter of this population. Hispanic children with families living in older houses also fell victims of elevated blood lead levels. Baltimore City is among the cities with the highest percentage of childhood lead poisoning prevalence (Zaleski, 2020). It may not surprise some childhood lead-based paint poison advocates that in 2018, ninety-nine (99) children were identified as clinically lead poisoned in Baltimore City (Ramos, 2018). If the policy had mandated property owners to perform lead abatement or other risk reduction measures, continued incidences of childhood lead poisoning could have been avoided by this time. The policy failed to assess the risk of lead-based paint or did not consider the consequences of lead exposure to children (Kassa, Bisesi, Khuder, & Park, 2000). In Baltimore City the trend of lead-based paint exposure and poisoning decreased with the help of local ordinance as shown in figure 6.3 between 1995 through 2006.

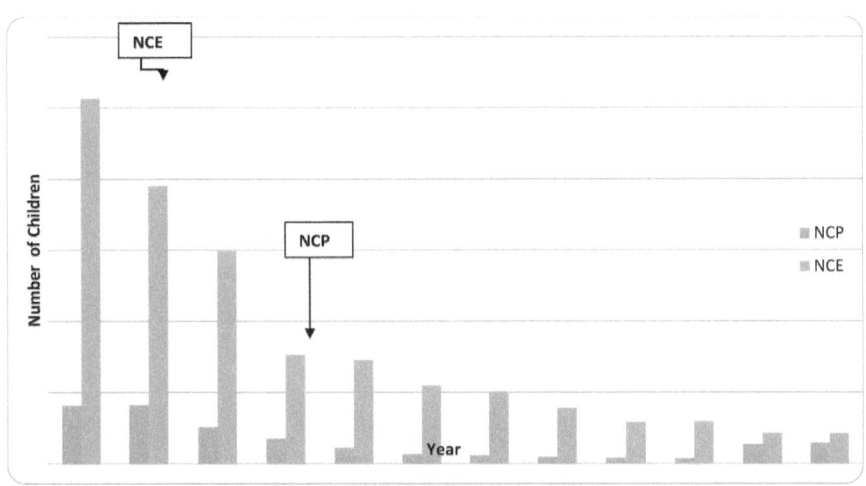

Source: Iregbu, 2008.

Figure 6.3: Trend in Childhood Lead-Based Paint Exposure and Poisoning in Baltimore City in Pre and Post the Disclosure Policy

Note: The Policy became effective on September 6, 1996. NCE=Number of children exposed; NCP= Number of children poisoned.

The federal Disclosure Policy on residential lead-based paint alone was not adequate to increase the number of lead abatements and risk-reduction measures. It has been more enforcement action through promulgation of state and local regulations of lead-based paint housing code in Baltimore City that increased lead abetment in the city older homes. More so, Maryland Department of the Environment (MDE) promulgated Environmental Article Title 6-Sect-819 (a), and on 28 February 2006, the Baltimore City Health Department published Abatement Regulation for Lead-Based Paint (Baltimore City, 2006). As the state and local laws became effectively implemented in Baltimore City, abatements and other lead risk-reduction measures improved in 2001(Iregbu, 2008).

Chapter 6 References:

1. Abell Foundation, (2002). Childhood lead poisoning in Baltimore: A generation imperiled as laws ignored. The Abell Report, 15 (5).
2. Agency for Toxic Substances and Disease Registry (ATSDR). (1997). Lead and your health. *ATSDR*, August, 1997.
3. Baltimore City Health Department, (2006). Abatement Regulation for Lead-Based Paint. Baltimore City Dept. of Health, 2006.
4. Images for Baltimore, (2006). Local Laws about Lead. Retrieved from http://www.leadsafehomes.com.
5. CDC, (1997). Screening young children for lead poisoning: Guidance for state and local public health officials (pp. 13-20). CDC, Atlanta, GA. Nov. 1997.
6. CDC, (2015). At-risk populations. Centers for Disease Control and Prevention (CDC) 2015. Retrievedfrom: http://www.cdc.gov/nceh/lead/tips/populations.htm.
7. Environmental Protection Agency (EPA), (1997). Lead-based paint abatement and repair and maintenance study in Baltimore. EPA/747/R-97/001. Retrieved from http://www.epa.gov.
8. Environmental Protection Agency [EPA] & Housing and Urban Development [HUD]. (1998). EPA & HUD real estate notification and disclosure law on residential lead-based paint: Questions and answers. HUD Office of Lead Hazard Control, Washington, DC 20410 and EPA Office of Pollution Prevention and Toxics, Washington, DC 20460, 1998, 109-124. Retrieved from http://www.epa.gov.
9. Environmental Protection Agency (EPA)-747-F-96-001, (1996). Interpretative guidance for the real estate community on the requirements for disclosure of information concerning lead-based paint in housing. EPA, Office of Pollution

Prevention and Toxics, Washington, DC 20460, 1996. Retrieved from http://www.epa.gov.

10. Environmental Protection Agency (EPA)., (1992). Disclosure Policy on Residential Lead-based Paint. Code of Federal Registry 40, 745.

11. Gould, B. E. (2009). Childhood Lead Poisoning: Conservative Estimates of the Social and Economic Benefits of Lead Hazard Control. Environ Health Perspect. (Research Children's Health), 2009 Jul; 117(7): 1162–1167. Published online 2009 Mar 31. doi: 10.1289/ehp.0800408. PMCID: PMC2717145, PMID: 19654928.

12. Hauptman, M., Bruccoleri, R. and Woolf, A.D. (2017). An Update on Childhood Lead Poisoning. Clin Pediatr Emerg Med, 2017 Sep; 18(3): 181–192. doi: 10.1016/j. cpem.2017.07.010.

13. Iregbu, C. A., (2008). Lead Paint Disclosure Policy: Implications for Eliminating Childhood Lead Exposure in Baltimore City, 2008, University of Michigan Publishers. Also: Barnes and Noble Published online July 2011.

14. Kassa, H., Bisesi, M. S., Khuder, S. A., & Park, P. C. (2000). Assessment of a lead management program for inner-city children. Journal of Environmental health, 62 (10), 15-35.

15. Miller, B.M.G, (2011). Practical guidelines for evaluating lead exposure in children with mental health conditions: molecular effects and clinical implications. Postgrad Med. 2011;123(1):160–8. [PubMed].

16. National Center for Environmental Health (NCEH), (2019). Lead Poisoning Prevention. NCEH; Division of Environmental Health Science and Practice. July 30, 2019.

17. Maryland Department of the Environment, (1999). Predictive Area of High Risk for Lead Poisoning in Baltimore City by Census Track with Zip Code Overlay for Children Under 6 Years of Age. MDE, 1999.

18. McCoy, T. (2015). Freddie Gray's life a study on the effects of lead paint on poor blacks The Washington Post, April 29, 2015.
19. Ramos, A. R. (2018). As Lead Poisoning Cases In Baltimore Rise, Group Hopes To Help Homeowners Remove Hazards. Baltimore, Baltimore News, Lead Paint, Lead Poisoning, Local TV, Talkers; December 13, 2019 at 5:37 pm.
20. US Environmental Protection Agency (USEPA)., (1992). Disclosure Policy on Residential Lead-based Paint. Code of Federal Registry 40, 745.
21. Wallerstein, N., Yen, I., and Syme, S. (2011). Integration of social epidemiology and community-engaged interventions to improve health equity. American Journal of Public Health, 101(5), 822-830.
22. Zaleski, A. (2020). The Unequal Burden of Urban Lead. Bloomberg CityLab. January 2, 2020.

CHAPTER 7

The Role of Epidemiology in Public Health–The COVID19 Pandemic Example

The Common Understanding

The effectiveness of a public health program is determined by process, implementation, impact and outcome evaluations of the program. These sequence of activities enable program planers, directors and stakeholders to make changes where necessary. The ultimate focus is to meeting the goal for which the program is designed. This concept transcends to application of evidenced-based policy and practice in public health promotion and health service delivery. Decision making process must employ evidence based concept to enhance maximum resources to better the health of the population. The role of research and scientific analysis in health policy decision making and health promotion is very important. It provides strategies in health management agenda in areas of intervention and other clinical decision making. For example, procedures, and practices that cause more harm than good can be stopped or slowed and vice versa (Muir-Gray, 2001). Epidemiology as a track in public health has elevated public awareness on most chronic diseases in terms of who is affected, potential causality factors and approach to mitigate impacts of diseases (Korff, 2011).

Science of Epidemiology and Public Health

It was the efforts of scientists that identified the novel coronavirus associated with a severe acute respiratory disease similar to pneumonia cases in Wuhan City, China. Relevant symptoms and data documented from people with the illness revealed a resemblance to Coronaviruses (CoVs) in the genus Coronavirus in *Coronaviridae* family (McIntosh, Hirsch & Bloom, 2020). When a disease occurs among a give population or region in a number that is far more than normal in the past cases and exhibiting strange symptoms, it is regarded as epidemic. This is where the science of epidemiology come to play a role. It invokes surveillance, documentation of demographical and analysis data related to the victims of the disease. It goes further to observe and monitor vehicle of spread or transmission of the disease, rate of incidences and mortality (Friis & Sellers, 2014). In addition epidemiology also attempt to identify groups of people or individuals at risk of getting infected during an outbreak of a new disease (Macera, Shaffer & Shaffer, 2013). Scientist work together with public health experts as in other times especially when there is a new disease outbreak. This was typical when the pneumonia related cases of disease in Wuhan City, China spread fast into other parts of mainland China and into other countries throughout the world.

It was on this frame of reference that global observation and surveillance became intensified to recognize that CoVs like symptoms and illness has spread into many global regions and continents. Based on these facts global epidemiologist and infectious disease experts agreed and categorized the illness as a **pandemic** (Dawood, et al., 2020). With this understanding and decision, the status of the pneumonia related cases of the disease in Wuhan City, China,

in late 2019 was officially declared as a pandemic by the World
Health Organization (WHO), (WHO, 2020). The disease was so
coined as COVID-19. This code name stand for coronavirus disease
2019. The work of epidemiology did not stop here rather the task of
documenting the number of deaths, active cases and how different
groups and individual respond to the disease become important in
understanding how to fight and mitigate the problem.

As the global cases increased with same severe acute respiratory
syndrome caused by coronavirus 2 (SARS-CoV-2), WHO started to
issue some guidelines on how to control the pandemic (Rettner, 2020).
Before the official upgrade of the disease, the United States Centre
for Disease Control (CDC) had already put it's epidemiological
machinery into action. This was by lunching the agency-wide
response preparedness on January 27, 2020. This included putting
first responders, healthcare providers, and health systems on alert
and ready for action (CDC, 2020).

This principle is the core reason why scientists around the world
scrambled and worked tirelessly around the clock as to find a cure
and or a measure to mitigate the danger of COVID19 on human
population. While the lay person is disturbed about the safety of
vaccine, scientists are optimistic that following evidenced-based
protocols, a safe vaccine with acceptable efficacy will likely be in the
market considering the rigorous time it takes for the actual production.
This optimism though must be checked applying standard of cost
benefit analysis and other risk factors that may be associated with the
potential product. For the meantime, epidemiologists have strongly
advised on evidence-based practises that help minimize person-
to-person transmission of the disease and infection. These include
adhering to personal hygiene of frequent washing of hands, avoiding
touching of mouth and nostrils, wearing of mask in the public places
with people and maintaining at least 6ft of social distancing.

What We Know About Developing a Vaccine

Vaccine research, testing and production is not a process of *garbage in garbage out*. In situation of new disease outbreak like Ebola and COVID19 pandemic, it involves all potential stakeholders to include various research groups from academia, industries and the government. Irrespective of the urgency that a new infectious disease outbreak impose on human population researchers and policy makers must not rush to approve a new vaccine. For example, the issues of use of Thimerosal in vaccines have been a long controversy. In one instance a two week time frame within which the responsible federal agencies had to work to develop a response to the Thimerosal in vaccine was very limited. With such time constrain it was obvious that adequate review of data, comparison of information and possibly independent clinical trial of the vaccine was not feasible.

Vaccines have actually reduced cases of most virulent infectious agents. Approval and administration of vaccines that prevented certain diseases such as *Polio* and *Small Pox* are commendable public health policy including COVID19 vaccines that were vigorously pursued, tested and approved by US food and drug administration (US-FDA) under emergency use. In the event that the use of a vaccine results into more morbidity and mortality due to a higher dose of the attenuating agent, such vaccine is then doing more harm than good. Most times some drugs and vaccines are recalled from the market and utilization after adverse side effects manifest among human consumers. One of the purposes and goal of scientific research is to enable the assessment of intervention strategies, promote better health and prevent illness through the use of data gathered during the investigation (Gray-Muir, 2001). Thereafter, information is presented as evidence for public health policy promotion and formation. No ethically rooted research scientist will like his or her work stained relative to public health services as it was compromised in the thimerosal issue (Freed et al, 2002).

Epidemiology and COVID19

During COVID19 pandemic daily briefings and updates by the White House Task Force on COVID19 in 2020, epidemiologists and other scientists threaded very carefully on questions to how soon a vaccine will be ready for COVID19. The disease is a new outbreak requiring more research and knowledge on how to diagnose and treat infected individuals. Most importantly is on how to break the cycle of infection known as epidemiological triangle (Friis, 2010). That is building a virtual wall between the primary host of the infecting agent or source, the rest of the environment and future potential victims (see Figure 7.1). Epidemiologists take investigation of new disease outbreak very serious. In so doing, investigations must ensure the source of the disease, the specific primary host of the infectious agent's mode of transmission, incubation period, symptoms and conditions that enable the infections agent thrive (Rourke & Roach, 2010). The CDC and the *COVID19 Task Force* were aware of these and as such worked towards providing authentic epidemiological data. Moreover, they must be mindful as to apply appropriate approach in terms of information dissemination out for the public consumption (CDC, COVID-19 Epidemiology, 2020). In this time and era of electronic information technology, the public is absolutely curious to know what is new relative to the pandemic. In addition to traditional television news, the public search for such desired information online using various and available electronic devices (Ripberger, 2011).

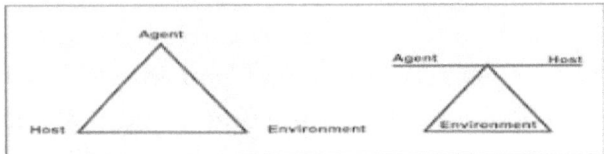

Figure 7.1: **Epidemiological Triangle**

In applying epidemiology in public health policy decision making, Braithwaite et al. (1999) stated that epidemiology cannot prove safety. Also, it cannot provide causation, ether generally or in a specific case. Hence the intension of the statement was to delineate the function of epidemiological studies from ethology and potentials of associable risk factors for diseases or harms that affect humans. In essence, the general public and non-scientists in particular should be educated on how different scientific research data and analysis can be utilized as evidence in decision making and public health policy formation.

According to Braithwaite et al (1999), epidemiology is the study of the distribution and determinants of disease in humans. If this holds as the boundaries of epidemiological studies, then it will basically try to identify types of diseases among any given population. It will also report on mortality and death related rate and cases of such disease using statistical analysis. In doing this, the goal of epidemiological studies is to provide information for decision making on diseases and other risks that affect human population. This then means that the information provided through epidemiological study does not automatically imply a provision for safety on such a disease or risk factor. Similarly, information and data provided from epidemiological study must not be construed as providing a causation of a disease or risk factor. Rather, it must be reviewed, analysed and weighed against economic, social and various environmental health determinants tagged to policies and other factors in policy formation.

The implication of this statement is that all stakeholders in the decision making and public health policy formation need to understand what is important and what is not for making important health policy decisions. These include the legislators, the policy makers other scientists as well as the epidemiologists. Epidemiologists have long viewed the field very important and has welcomed the notion that epidemiology is the foundation of public health science as epidemiological data measures risk directly in human. However, such measurements are the most relevant indicators of adverse effect in humans (Matanoski, 2001). Nonetheless, epidemiological studies have also been criticized as being just observed studies without a control group like toxicological studies. Besides that, in presenting epidemiological data for potential usage in policy formation, the epidemiologist must minimize the use of complicated statistical analysis. It must not act as advocate, rather should act as a presenter of information. The epidemiologist must also be ready and willing to answer complex questions and clarify ambiguous statements. This stand manifested very much in 2020 during the White House Daily Briefing on COVID19. The epidemiologist must also try to understand both environmental and other regulations that may involve the use of epidemiological studies for policy decisions (Matanoski, 2001). On the other hand, public policy makers need to realize that neglecting evidence-based facts that support epidemiological recommendations is of high risk for public health.

The role of epidemiology plaid well with COVID19 case mortality. It is very important to reflect on specific population that were mostly affected and the environment surrounding such particular population. In addition to African American minority, the elderly in nursing homes suffered a greater share of COVID19 mortality rate (Gebeloff et al., 2020). Why is it so, is a lesson we can learn from Werner, Rita & Kim (2013). As the COVID19 pandemic arrived into the United States, the early epidemiological data relating that the elderly are more susceptible to the disease, should have alerted nursing homes operators to develop and adopt quick and urgent quality measures. Such strategic measures would have improved patient outcomes and reduced the death rate in nursing homes.

Though appropriately recognised as pandemic, COVID19 has been often referred to as a disaster in the United States. When a disaster occurs, epidemiology also do study the pattern of morbidity and mortality. It also attempt to identify the causality and rate of fatality relative to each disaster. Furthermore, it draws relevant and comparable factors from past occurrences. The studies so far documented and published on COVID19 disaster has also implicated a vivid racial and ethnic bias in terms of adverse impacts (Cunningham, et al, 2017) and (Hall, et al, 2015). Evidence-based studies in epidemiology also focus on demographical variables to include social status and health literacy. A population with better understanding of healthy life style and living seem to be more cautious on how to react and adapt in times of possible disaster. Hence, the lower social status of a community tend to enable vulnerable conditions in time of a disaster (Thomas, Phillips, Lovekamp & Fothergill, 2013). According to Bolin, Bob, and Kurtz (2018) the less affluent are most likely to be vulnerable during disasters.

REFERENCES:

1. Braithwaite, W., Cole, P., Feinstein, A. R., Green, M., Hirsch, R., Lather, C. M., et al. (1999). The role of epidemiology in decision-making. Retrieved from http://www.annapoliscenter.org.
2. Bolin, Bob, and Liza C. Kurtz. "Race, class, ethnicity, and disaster vulnerability." Handbook of disaster research. Springer, Cham, 2018. 181–203.
3. CDC, (2020). CDC's Coronavirus Disease 2019 (COVID-19) Response, August 31, 2020. Extracted on September 1, 2020 from: https://www.cdc.gov/coronavirus/2019-ncov/cdcresponse/index.html.
4. CDC, (2020) About COVID-19 Epidemiology; Investigating COVID-19: The Science Behind CDC's Response. Extracted on August 31, 2020; from: https://www.cdc.gov/coronavirus/2019-ncov/cases-updates/about-epidemiology/index.html, July 1, 2020.
5. Cunningham, T. J., Croft, J. B., Liu, Y., Lu, H., Eke, P. I., & Giles, W. H. (2017). Vital signs: racial disparities in age-specific mortality among blacks or African Americans—United States, 1999–2015. MMWR. Morbidity and mortality weekly report, 66(17), 444.
6. Dawood, et al. (2020). Observations of the global epidemiology of COVID-19 from the pre-pandemic period using web-based

surveillance: a cross-sectional analysis. Extracted August 29, 2020 from: https://www.thelancet.com/journals/laninf/article/PIIS1473-3099(20)30581-8/fulltext. DOI: https://doi.org/10.1016/S1473-3099(20)30581-8.Elsevier Ltd. ScienceDirect.

7. Freed, G. L. et al. (2001). The process of public policy formulation: The case of thimerosal in vaccines. Pediatrics, Vol 109 (6).

8. Friis, R. H., & Sellers, T. (2014). Epidemiology for public health practice (5th ed.). Burlington, MA: Jones & Bartlett Learning.

9. Friis, R. H. (2010). Epidemiology 101. Sudbury, MA: Jones & Bartlett Learning.

10. Gebeloff et al., (2020). The Striking Racial Divide in How Covid-19 Has Hit Nursing Homes. The New York Times, May 21, 2020.

11. Hall et al., (2015). Implicit Racial/Ethnic Bias Among Health Care Professionals and Its Influence on Health Care Outcomes: A Systematic Review. *American journal of public health*, *105*(12), e60–e76. https://doi.org/10.2105/AJPH.2015.302903.

12. Macera, C. A., Shaffer, R., & Shaffer, P. M. (2013). Introduction to epidemiology: Distribution and determinants of disease (1st ed.). Clifton Park, NY: Cengage Learning.

13. Matanoski, G., (2001). Conflicts between two cultures: Implications for epidemiologic researchers in communicating with policy-makers. American Journal of Epidemiology, Vol.154, No.12, S36-S42.

14. McIntosh, K.; Hirsch, M.S. and Bloom, A. (2020). Coronavirus disease 2019 (COVID-19): Epidemiology, virology, and prevention. Wolters Kluwer UpToDate; Extracted from:

15. Muir Gray, J.A, (2001). Evidenced-based healthcare: How to make health policy and management decisions (2nd ed) Edinburg: Churchill Livingstone, p37-62.

16. O'Rourke, K. M. and Roach, M. (2010). Disease Investigation. (2nd ed.). Edgewater, FL: DLK Publishing.

17. Rettner, R. (2020). Coronavirus outbreak officially declared a pandemic, WHO says. Extracted August 30, 2020. from: https://www.livescience.com/coronavirus-pandemic-who. html, March 11, 2020.

18. Ripberger, J. (2011). Capturing curiosity: Using Internet search trends to measure public attentiveness. Policy Studies Journal, 39(2), 239-259.

19. Thomas, D.S., Phillips, B.D., Lovekamp, W.E. and Fothergill, A., 2013. Social vulnerability to disasters. CRC Press.

20. Werner, R. M., Rita, T., & Kim, M. (2013). Quality improvement under nursing home compare: the association between changes in process and outcome measures. Med Care. 5197, 582-8.

21. WHO, (2020). Emergencies preparedness, response: pneumonia of unknown cause—China. Extracted August 30, 2020, from: https://www.who.int/csr/don/05-january-2020-pneumonia-of-unkown-cause-china/en/; Jan 5, 2020.

22. Korff, V. M. (2011). Public health approaches to chronic pain: the role of epidemiology. The Lancet Neurology, 10(3), 210-211.

Appedix—A

Appendix A: Sample Socio-Economic and Racial/Ethnic Distribution in Baltimore City Neighborhood with Population ≥ 2000 Persons.

Neighborhood/(Economic Rating)	Population	Zip Code	W (%)	B (%)*
Allendale (2)	84	229	.6	98.1
Arlington (2)	3,055	21214	2.4	94.9
Armistead Gardens (-)	2,911	21214	92.0	.02
Ashburton (1)	3,055	21215	.01	95.80
Baltimore Highlands (2)	2,313	21224	66.1	25.91
Barclay (2)	2,718	21224	.07	90.05
Beechfield (2)	3,758	21229/8	14.0	83.1
Belair-Edison (2)	16,523	21213	19.1	77.9
Berea (2)	4,525	21213	.01	98.32
Better Waverly (2)	2,573	21218	14.26	81.03
Bolton Hill (1)	5,292	21217	59.5	32.5
Bridgeview/ Greenlawn (2)	2,310	21216	.002	98.65
Broadway East (2)	6,836	21213	.001	98.12
Brooklyn (2)	8,031	21225	74.82	18.24
Canton (1)	10,887	21214	91.73	.03
Carrolton Ridge (2)	3,525	21223	48.54	45.0
Cedmont (1)	2,581	21206	75.7	21.4
Cedonia (2)	3,581	21206	10.63	87.12
Central Park Heights (2)	7,865	21215	.96	97.89
Charles Village (1)	6,549	21218	58.8	25.5

Cherry Hill (2)	7,801	21225	2.96	95.71
Cheswolde (1)	6,361	21209	82.50	12.29
Chinquapin Park-Belvedere (1)	2,111	21212	22.69	74.51
Coldstream/Homestead/ Montebello (2)	8,737	21218	1.16	97.0
Coppin Heights/Ash-Co-East (2)	3,104	21216	.93	98.26
Cross Country (1)	4,114	21215/08/09	85.03	11.64
Curtis Bay (2)	3,983	21226	76.87	17.9
Cylburn (2)	2,586	21215	.85	98.03
Dolfield (2)	2,243	21215	.71	98.13
Downtown (1)	3,177	21201/2	44.38	41.99
East Balt. Midway (2)	4,139	21218	1.28	96.45
Edmondson Village (2)	7,092	21229	.49	98.03
Ednor Gardens-LakeSide (1)	5,200	21218	15.71	81.34
Ellwood Park/Monument (2)	4,489	21205	16.6	79.0
Falls Staff (1)	4,108	21215/08	45.57	47.66
Federal Hill-Montgomery (1)	2,274	21230	87.2	8.5
Fells Point (1)	4,13,049	2121231	79.7	9.2
Fifteenth Street (-)	2,174	-	80.6	5.7
Frankford (2)	16,792	21206	22.9	74.1
Franklin Square (2)	3,536	21223	1.9	96.1

Neighborhood/(Economic Rating)	Population	Zip code	W (%)	B (%)*
Gay Street (2)	2,083	21216	1.0	97.5
Glen (1)	8,938	21215/6	43.8	52.1
Glen Oaks (1)	2,932	21239	15.6	79.6
Glenham-Belford (1)	6,089	21206	67.1	29.3
Green Spring (2)	4,049	21215	1.1	98.1
Grove Park (1)	2,095	21215/07	0.67	96.8
Guilford (1)	2,098	21210/18	80.8	13.4
Hampden (1)	8,089	21211	93.5	2.80
Hanlon-Longwood (2)	2,689	21216	0.37	98.4
Harford-Echodale /Perring Parkway (-)	8,475	-	32.5	64.0
Harlem Park (2)	4,719	21223/17	0.4	98.4
Harwood (2)	2,105	21218	7.6	89.07
Highlandtown (1)	2,821	21224	77.5	11.8
Hillen (1)	2,809	21218	6.9	90.1
Hollins Market (1)	2,050	21223	33.9	59.3

Neighborhood/(Economic Rating)	Population	Zip code	W (%)	B (%)*
Homeland (1)	3,088	21212	88.1	8.5
Howard Park (1)	6,045	21207	2.4	95.5
Idlewood (1)	2,710	21239	26.3	69.5
Irvington (2)	4,401	21229	14.9	82.4
Johnston Square (2)	2,727	21202	1.6	97.2
Joseph Lee (1)	2,176	21224	86.1	4.4
Lake Walker (1)	2,085	21212	58.4	35.2
Lakeland (2)	4,280	21230	42.2	53.4
Lauraville (1)	4,375	21214	51.47	43.74
Loch Raven (1)	6,136	21239	16.3	80.1
Locust Point (1)	2,208	21230	97.19	0.58
Loyola/NotreDame (1)	4,072	21212	82.1	12.5
Madison Pak (1)	2,140	21217	9.6	86.9
Madison-East End (2)	2,457	21205	4.5	93.0
McElderry Park (2)	3,476	21205	10.1	86.1
Medfield (1)	2,760	21211	80.6	12.4
Medford/Broening- Manor (1)	2,725	21224	67.0	21.46
Mid-Govans (2)	2,373	21212	16.3	80.4
Mid-Town Belvedere (1)	3,194	21202	53.7	35.6
Middle East (2)	4,921	21205	3.1	94.5
Midtown Edmondson (2)	2,328	21216/7	0.34	98.8
Mondawmin (2)	3,556	21216/7	0.53	98.0
MorrelPark (2)	4,727	21230	93.0	3.22
Mosher (2)	2,009	21216	0.29	99.0
Mount Clare (2)	2,393	21223	55.83	38.91
Mount Vernon (1)	3,192	21201/2	58.1	30.58
Mount Washington (1)	3,637	21209/15	80.23	16.68
New Northwood (2)	6,863	21239	2.14	96.46
North Harford Road (1)	5,281	21234	80.85	15.09
N.W. Community −Action (2)	2,088	21216	0.43	98.75
Neighborhood/(Economic Rating)	Population	Zip code	W (%)	B (%)*
O'Donnell Heights (2)	2,217	21224	18.0	77.36
Oakenshawe (1)	2,457	21216	65.21	12.49
Oliver (2)	5473	21202/13	0.62	98.37
Park Circle (2)	3,833	21215	0.97	96.09
Parklane (2)	2,129	21215	1.46	96.20
Parkside (2)	2,549	21206	10.36	87.13
Parkview/Wallbrook (2)	2,334	21217	0.60	97.73
Patterson Park (2)	5,955	21214	42.63	46.0

Pen Lucy (2)	3,265	21218	5.79	90.34
Penn North (2)	2,342	21217	0.68	97.36
Penn-Fallsway (-)	7.208	-	12.3	87.61
Penrose (2)	3,353	21223	0.26	98.39
Perring Loch (1)	3,122	21234	8.5	89.49
Poppleton (1)	2,869	21223/01	2.4	96.23
Ramblewood (1)	2,020	21239	9.7	86.98
Remington (2)	2,308	21211	59.5	31.76
Reservoir Hill (1)	6,901	21217	6.54	91.39
Riverside (1)	5,564	21230	94.73	2.25
Rognel Heights (2)	2,154	21229	1.11	97.31
Roland Park (1)	3,577	21210	89.24	5.12
Rosemont (2)	3,129	21216	0.32	97.82
Saint Josephs (2)	2,269	21229	1.85	96.09
Sandtown-Winchester (2)	9,254	21217	**0.68**	**97.68**
South Baltimore (SBIC) (1)	3,915	21230	89.20	7.08
Seton Hill (1)	2,143	21201	16.19	75.78
Shipley Hill (2)	2,454	21223	4.02	95.16
Tuscany-Canterbury (1)	3,447	21210/18	78.60	0.50
Uplands (2)	2,523	21229	1.98	96.99
Upper Fells Point (1)	4,840	21231	75.10	8.44
Upton (2)	4,509	21217	0.71	97.92
Violetvill (1)	2,677	21227/9	91.52	5.67
Walbrook (2)	2,810	21216	1.81	96.33
Waltherson (1)	5,907	21214	54.95	40.92
Washington Hill (1)	2,404	21231	21.09	71.13
Washington Village (2)	5,410	21230	48.81	44.77
Waverly (2)	3,175	21218	11.65	84.44
West Arlington (1)	2,273	21215	1.21 9	6.29
West Forest Park (2)	2,532	21216	3.63	94.71
West Hills (2)	2,157	21229	9.92	88.04
Westfield (1)	2,721	21214	77.51	18.85
Westgate (1)	2,874	21229/8	34.12	62.77
Winchester (2)	2,083	21216	0.53	98.17
Woodmere (2)	2,308	21216	1.82	96.03
Woodring (1)	2,488	21234	84.0	13.82
Yale Heights (1)	2,891	21229	10.65	87.75

Source: Iregbu (2008).Table generated from BCDP City's 2000 Census Population by Race and Neighborhood.(1) = Affluent, (2) = non-affluent, (-) no category, W= White, B=Black, (* % Hispanic, Native American, Asian and Other Races were all very small and did not constitute dominant race in any neighborhood.